U0332570

英文原版

Blepharoplasty

Thomas Procedures in Facial Plastic Surgery

Thomas 面部美容整形：眼睑成形术

Ira D. Papel, MD, FACS
Facial Plastic Surgicenter
Associate Professor
The Johns Hopkins University
Baltimore, Maryland, USA

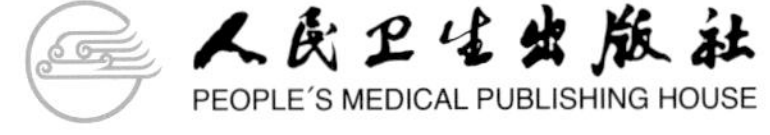

English reprinted edition of Thomas Procedures in FACIAL PLASTIC SURGERY: Blepharoplasty by Ira D. Papel

The original English language work has been published by People's Medical Publishing House-USA, Ltd.
© 2012 PMPH-USA, Ltd.

Reprinted by People's Medical Publishing House
© 2017 People's Medical Publishing House
Beijing, China

图书在版编目（CIP）数据

Thomas 面部美容整形．眼睑成形术：英文 /（美）艾拉·D.·帕佩（Ira D. Papel）主编．—北京：人民卫生出版社，2017

ISBN 978-7-117-25771-8

Ⅰ．① T…　Ⅱ．①艾…　Ⅲ．①眼睑－整形外科学－英文　Ⅳ．① R622

中国版本图书馆 CIP 数据核字（2017）第 312300 号

人卫智网	www.ipmph.com	医学教育、学术、考试、健康，购书智慧智能综合服务平台
人卫官网	www.pmph.com	人卫官方资讯发布平台

版权所有，侵权必究！

Thomas 面部美容整形：眼睑成形术（英文版）

主　　编：Ira D. Papel
出版发行：人民卫生出版社（中继线 010-59780011）
地　　址：北京市朝阳区潘家园南里 19 号
邮　　编：100021
E - mail：pmph @ pmph.com
购书热线：010-59787592　010-59787584　010-65264830
印　　刷：北京盛通印刷股份有限公司
经　　销：新华书店
开　　本：787 × 1092　1/16　　印张：8.5
字　　数：207 千字
版　　次：2017 年 12 月第 1 版　2017 年 12 月第 1 版第 1 次印刷
标准书号：ISBN 978-7-117-25771-8/R・25772
定　　价：109.00 元
打击盗版举报电话：010-59787491　E-mail：WQ @ pmph.com
（凡属印装质量问题请与本社市场营销中心联系退换）

Contributors

Sumit Bapna, MD
Chief Resident
Department of Otolaryngology - Head and Neck Surgery
The Ohio State University
Columbus, OH

Kofi Boahene, MD
Assistant Professor
Facial Plastic and Reconstructive Surgery
Otolaryngology Head and Neck Surgery
Johns Hopkins University School of Medicine
Baltimore, MD

Eugene A. Chu, MD
Otolaryngology Head and Neck Surgery
Johns Hopkins University School of Medicine
Baltimore, MD

Christopher R Cote, MD
Board Certified and Fellowship Trained Facial Plastic and Reconstructive Surgery
Board Certified Otolaryngology/Head & Neck Surgery
Faces First Cosmetic Surgery
Denver, CO

Lisa A. Earnest, MD
Assistant Professor
Division of Facial Plastic and Reconstructive Surgery
Department of Otolaryngology-Head and Neck Surgery
The Johns Hopkins University
Baltimore, MD

Marc J. Hirschbein, MD, FACS
Associate Chairman
The Krieger Eye Institute
Sinai Hospital of Baltimore
Director,
The Center for Advanced Aesthetic Eyelid and Facial Surgery Division of Oculoplastic Surgery
Baltimore, MD

James Karesh, MD
Director of Oculoplastic Surgery
The Krieger Eye Institute
Sinai Hospital of Baltimore
Baltimore, MD

Theda C. Kontis, MD, FACS
Facial Plastic Surgeon
Facial Plastic Surgicenter
Assistant Professor
Johns Hopkins Medical Institutions
Baltimore, MD

Samuel M. Lam, MD
Director
Willow Bend Wellness Center
Lam Facial Plastic Surgery Center & Hair Restoration Institute
Plano, TX

Guy G. Massry, MD
Director
Ophthalmic Plastic and Reconstructive Surgery
Spalding Drive Cosmetic Surgery and Dermatology
Beverly Hills, CA

Paul S. Nassif, MD, FACS
Clinical Assistant Professor
Department of Otolaryngology –
Head & Neck Surgery
Division of Facial Plastic & Reconstructive Surgery
University of California – Los Angeles School of Medicine
Los Angles and University of Southern California, CA

Ira D. Papel, MD, FACS
Facial Plastic Surgicenter
Associate Professor
The Johns Hopkins University
Baltimore, MD

Stephen P. Smith, Jr., MD
Medical Director
Smith Facial Plastics
Dublin, OH
Director
Division of Facial Plastic and Reconstructive Surgery
Assistant Professor
Department of Otolaryngology-Head and Neck Surgery
The Ohio State University
Columbus, OH

Ifepo O. Sofola, MD, FACS
CEO
Inkerra Facial Plastics and Rhinology
Houston, TX

Edwin F. Williams, III, MD
Facial Plastic and Reconstructive Surgery
Williams Center for Excellence
Latham, NY
Facial Plastic and Reconstructive Surgery
Department of Surgery
Division of Otolaryngology-Head and Neck Surgery
Albany Medical Center
Albany, NY

Table of Contents

1

Surgical Anatomy of the Eyelid

Eugene A. Chu, MD, Theda C. Kontis, MD and Ira D. Papel, MD

Introduction

The eyes are the most prominent facial feature and provide important cues for recognition and emotion. The eyelids serve a critical function by protecting the anterior surface of the globe from dessication and local trauma. Furthermore, they aid in tear film maintenance, and their movement distributes the tear film evenly as it makes it way to the medial canthus to enter the lacrimal system. Blepharoplasty is an important component of the surgical treatment of the aging face and understanding the detailed anatomy of the eyelid is critical to its success.

The eyelids are multilamellar structures divided into an anterior lamella containing skin and orbicularis oculi muscle and a posterior lamella composed of the tarsal plate and conjunctiva (**Figure 1-1**). This chapter reviews key structures of lid anatomy: skin and subcutaneous tissues, orbicularis oculi muscle, submuscular areolar tissue, tarsal plates, lid margins, orbital septum, preapneurotic fat pads, lid retractors, and conjunctiva. Additionally, the neurovascular anatomy and relevant related surgical anatomy will be discussed.

Surface Anatomy

The upper and lower eyelids (palpebrae) are folds of tissue that meet at the medial and lateral aspects of the globe at each canthus. The upper lid extends superiorly to the eyebrow, whereas the lower lid merges with the cheek below the inferior orbital rim. The lateral canthus lies 2 to 4 mm superior to the medial canthus. While the lids are open, they form an elliptical space—the palpebral fissure—which is approximately 10–12 mm high and 28–30 mm wide (**Figure 1-2**). With age, height may decrease to only 8–10 mm.

The surface of the eyelid and periorbital region has multiple folds and mounds that are visible (**Figure 1-2**). The superior palpebral sulcus is formed by the attachment of the levator aponeurotic fibers to the skin of the upper eyelid and is located approximately 8–11 mm superior to the eyelid margin. The inferior palpebral sulcus, which is more prominent in children, is seen 3–6 mm below the lower lid margin and roughly delineates the inferior edge of the tarsal plate and the transition zone from pretarsal to preseptal orbicularis oculi. The nasojugal fold runs inferolaterally from the medial canthal region forming the so called tear trough. The adjacent malar fold is oriented inferomedially from the lateral canthus toward the inferior aspect of the nasojugal fold.

Eyelid Skin and Subcutaneous Tissue

The skin of the eyelids, measuring less than 1 mm in thickness, is the thinnest in the body. It is largely devoid of hair as well as subcutaneous fat. The epidermis lacks blood vessels and lymphatics, instead receiving its nutrients from a deeper layer of connective tissue—the corium. Just deep to the corium lays a very thin layer of subcutaneous loose connective tissues. The thin, delicate skin of the eyelid transitions to thicker, coarser skin as it extends beyond the superior lateral orbital rim and as it merges into the cheek. These textural differences should be considered in reconstructive surgery.

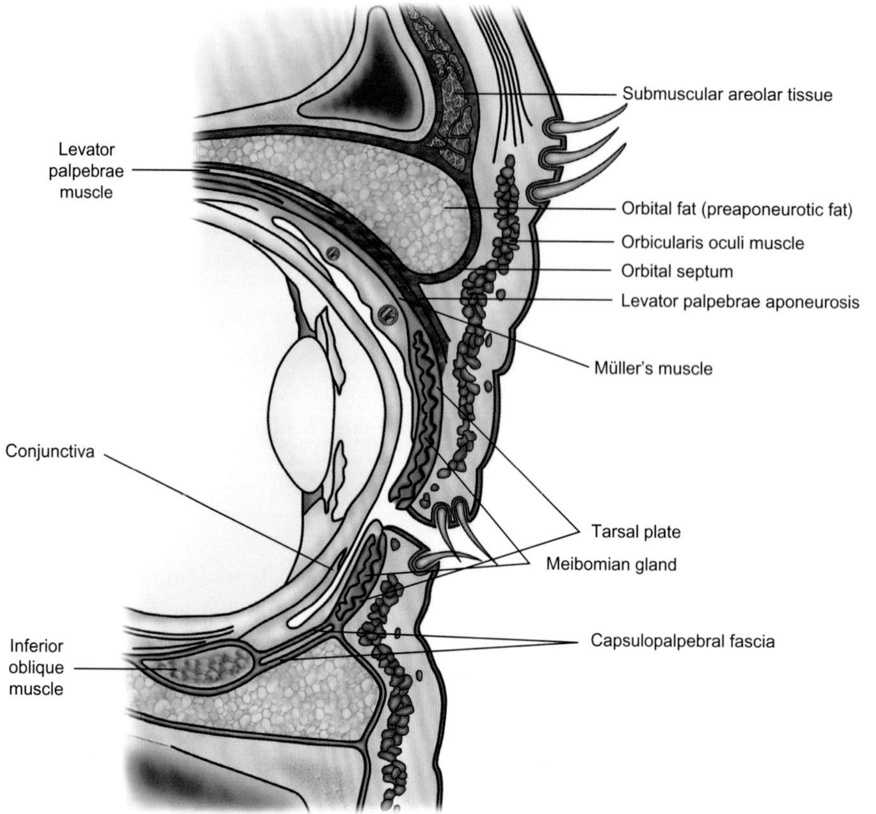

Figure 1-1. Sagittal section of the eyelid through the midpupillary line demonstrating its multilamellar structure.

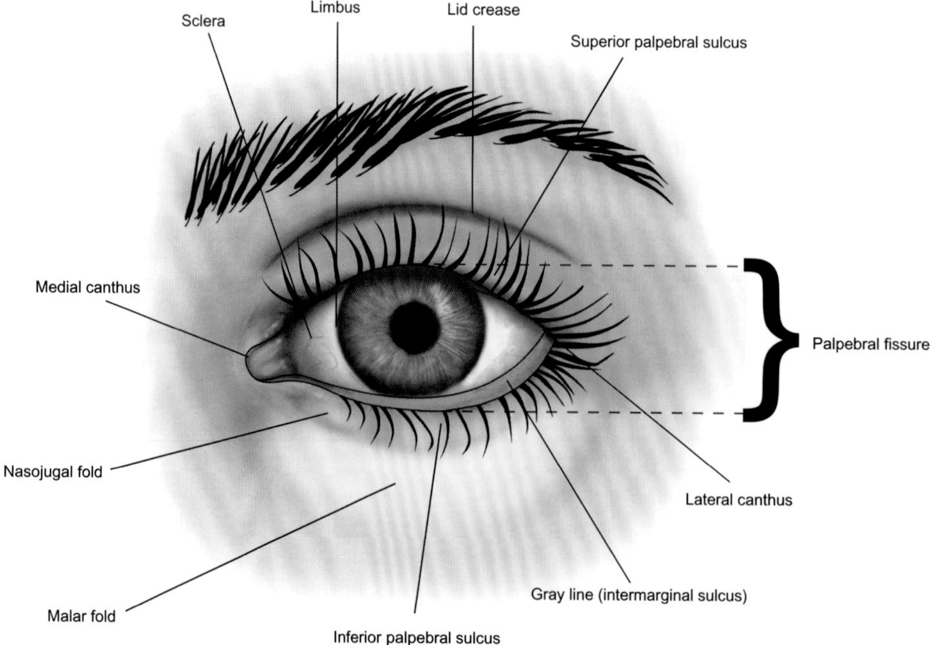

Figure 1-2. External landmarks of the eyelids and orbital region (left eye).

Orbicularis Oculi Muscle

The orbicularis oculi muscle is a complex striated muscle sheet deep to the skin and subcutaneous tissue of the eyelids. It is divided into two contiguous parts (orbital and palpebral) based on the region it overlies. The orbital portion is formed by concentric loops of muscle fibers that originate at the medial canthal tendon and travel around the orbital rim. Its action is to close the eyes tightly as in squinting. This portion of the muscle is generally not encountered during routine blepharoplasty surgery.

The palpebral portion extends from medial canthus to lateral canthus and can be further divided into preseptal and pretarsal components which overlie the orbital septum and tarsal plates respectively (**Figure 1-3**). Both divisions originate from two heads at the medial canthus. The superficial head of the preseptal and pretarsal portion arise from the medial canthal tendon, whereas the deep head of the preseptal division is attached to the posterior lacrimal crest and the deep head of the tarsal division to Horner's muscle (tensor tarsi). The muscle fibers of the preseptal component insert along the lateral horizontal raphe. The pretarsal fibers arc around the eyelids and insert onto the lateral canthal tendon and raphe. Contraction of these fibers aid in the lacrimal pump mechanism.

During blepharoplasty, conservative resection of the orbicularis oculi muscle is common. Overzealous resection can lead to loss of the muscular contractions necessary to move the tear film medially to the lacus lacrimalis. Additionally, inadvertent removal of tissue deep to the muscle can result in injury to the levator aponeurosis and subsequent ptosis. Careful dissection with identification of each anatomic layer will circumvent such injuries.

Submuscular Areolar Tissue

Just deep to the orbicularis oculi muscle lays the submuscular areolar tissue (**Figure 1-1**). These gossamer fibers are contiguous with the subaponeurotic layer of the scalp. The potential plane of the submuscular areolar tissue, which is accessed by division at the gray line (**Figure 1-2**) of the lid margin, separates the eyelid into an anterior and posterior portion. In the upper lid, this plane contains fibers of the levator aponeurosis as they pass through the orbicularis to attach to the skin forming the lid crease. As previously mentioned, injury to these fibers during blepharoplasty results in ptosis. Continuing superiorly in the same plane leads to the retro-orbicularis oculi fat (ROOF). Analogously, the lower lid potential plane is traversed by fibers of the orbitomalar ligament and is continuous inferiorly with the suborbicularis oculi fat (SOOF).

Tarsal Plates

The tarsal plates are the main supporting structures of the eyelid and are composed of dense fibrous connective tissue and a small amount of elastic tissue. The upper lid tarsus, which extends from the

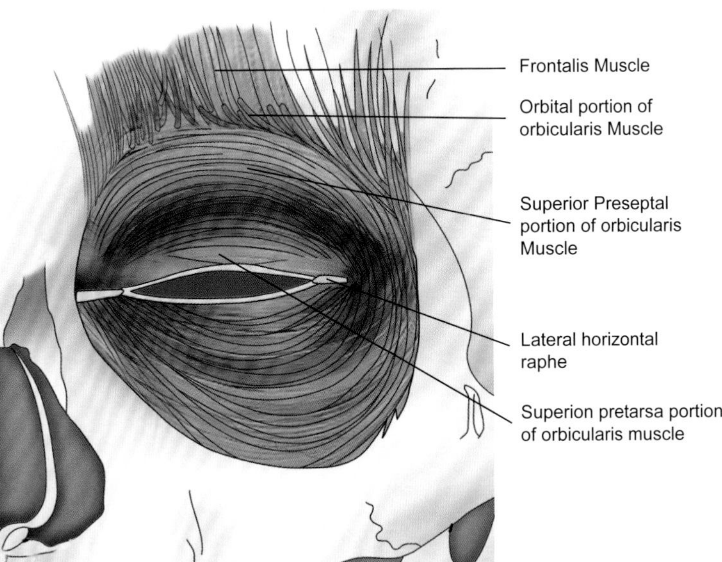

Figure 1-3. The subdivisions of the orbicularis oculi muscle and its relationship to medial canthal structures.

punctum to the lateral canthus, is approximately 30 mm long and 10 mm wide at its center. The lower tarsus is similar in length to the upper plate but only half as wide. Both plates are widest at the center, tapering at both ends. The plates contain grooves along their ciliary borders in which some 25 sebaceous meibomian glands can be found spanning the vertical height of the tarsus (**Figure 1-1**). The medial and lateral ends of the tarsi are attached to the orbital rims though the medial and lateral palpebral tendons (medial and lateral canthal tendons).

The medial canthal tendon (MCT), the medial extension of the fibrous tarsal plate, lies between the orbicularis muscle anteriorly and conjunctiva posteriorly. The superior and inferior crura fuse to form a common tendon that inserts into the orbit through three limbs (anterior, posterior, superior). The lateral canthal tendon (LCT), similarly formed by dense fibrous tissue arising from the tarsi, passes laterally deep to the orbital septum and inserts into the lateral orbital tubercle 1.5 mm posterior to the lateral orbital rim. The LCT is distinct from the orbicularis oculi muscle and is approximately 1 mm thick, 3 mm wide, and 5–7 mm long.

Lid Margins

The free lid margin is approximately 25–30 mm long and 2 mm wide. The gray line (mucocutaneous junction) partitions it into anterior and posterior margins. The anterior margins contains the eyelashes, glands of Zeis and Moll (sebaceous glands). The posterior margin is in contact with the globe and also contains sebaceous glands—tarsal glands along the lid margin.

Septum

The orbital septum is a fibrous connective tissue structure that represents the continuation of the periosteum from the orbital margin (the arcus marginalis) (**Figure 1-4A**). It lies just beneath the orbicularis muscle between the tarsus and orbital rim and functions as a partition between the lid and orbital contents. It is also an important anatomic landmark separating the orbit into an anterior and posterior compartment. Functionally, the septum acts as a barrier to infection and hemorrhage. With aging, the septum—which lies superficial to the orbital fat pads—weakens, allowing the prolapse of preaponeurotic fat (**Figure 1-4B**).

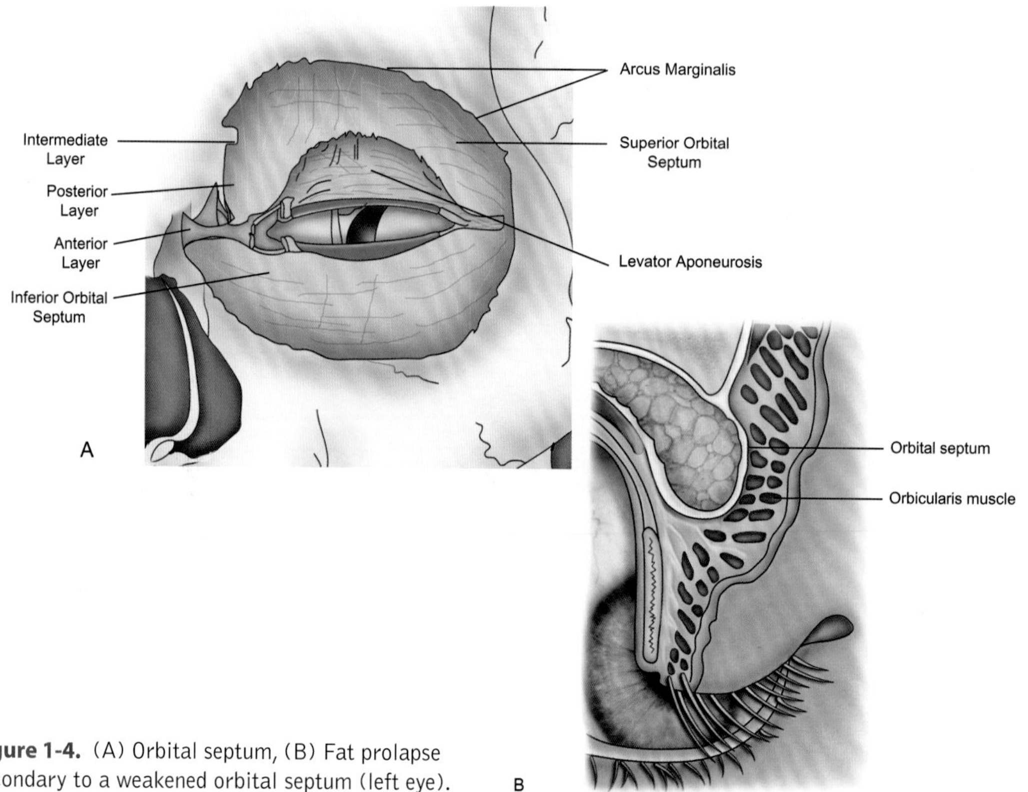

Figure 1-4. (A) Orbital septum, (B) Fat prolapse secondary to a weakened orbital septum (left eye).

Although the thickness of the septum varies, it is generally thicker laterally where it lies superficial to the LCT. Medially, the septum passes in front of the trochlea of the superior oblique muscle. Inferiorly, the orbital septum of the upper lid meets the levator aponeurosis approximately 2–5 mm above the tarsal plate (except in the eyelid of a person of Asian descent). The septum does not extend over the superficial aspect of the tarsal plates.

In the lower lid, approximately 5 mm inferior to the tarsus, the orbital septum joins the capsulopalpebral fascia—the anatomic analogue of the levator aponeurosis. Medially, the septum attaches to the anterior and posterior lacrimal crest and blends laterally with the LCT.

Preaponeurotic Fat Pads

The preaponeurotic fat pads are among the most important landmarks in eyelid surgery. They represent the anterior extension of extraconal orbital fat (**Figure 1-1**) and identify a plane immediately posterior to the orbital septum and anterior to the major eyelid retractors. Their distinctive color and location helps to guide dissection in revision surgery, when distinction between orbital septum and levator aponeurosis may be difficult.

Classically, two fat compartments are identified in the upper lid—medial and central. The lacrimal gland fills the lateral compartment of the upper lid and at times may be mistaken for a third fat pocket. However, several authors have recently reported the presence of a third, accessory, fat pad that was identified in about 20% of cases and located lateral to the central fat pad extending under the inferior border of the lacrimal gland (**Figure 1-5**). In both the upper and lower lids, the medial compartment is filled with a white, more fibrous fat pad. The central pad is usually pale yellow or white, whereas the lacrimal gland appears pinkish and is firm and lobulated in structure. The upper lid fat pads are separated by fascial strands arising from Whitnall's ligament. This white fibrous band extends from the lacrimal gland fascia to the trochlea, traveling parallel and superior to the levator aponeurosis. The ligament both suspends the globe and allows for changes in the direction of levator pull-up acting as a fulcrum.

In contrast to the upper lid, the lower lid has three compartments: medial, central, and lateral (**Figure 1-5**). The inferior oblique muscle separates the medial and central compartment and can be injured

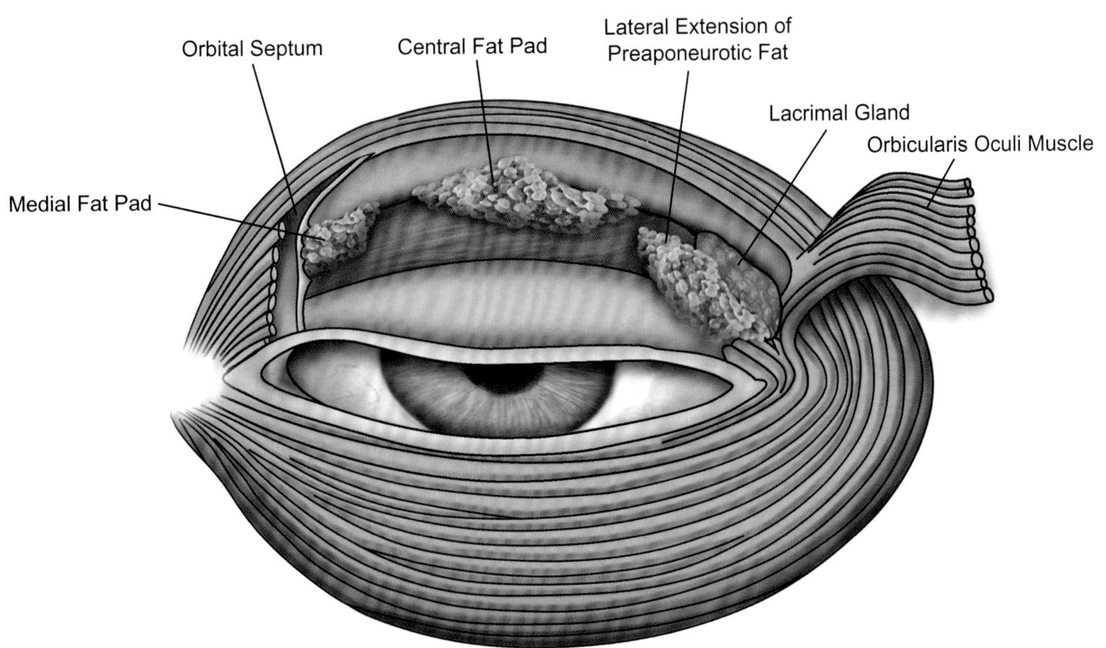

Figure 1-5. Adipose compartments of the upper and lower lid (left eye). This figure depicts the occasional occurrence of a lateral extension of preaponeurotic fat beneath the lacrimal gland.

during indiscriminant removal of the medial fat pad. Anatomic variants of the extent of compartmentalization have been reported and include the medial and lateral compartments positioned inferior to the central compartment, only two compartments, and loss of compartmentalization altogether. Nevertheless, the appearance of all three compartments side by side remains the common presentation.

Relatively large blood vessels supply the fat pads. Meticulous hemostasis is imperative during blepharoplasty to avoid retro-orbital hematomas and the potential for permanent ocular injury and blindness.

Lid Retractors

Lid retractors open the eyelids and are formed by a musculofascial complex with striated and smooth muscle components known as the levator complex in the upper lid and the capsulopalpebral fascia in the lower lid (**Figure 1-6**).

Upper Lid Retractors

The retractors of the upper lid consist of the levator palpebrae and Müller's muscle (**Figures 1-1 and 1-6**). The levator palpebrae superioris muscle is the primary elevator of the upper eyelid and is innervated by the oculomotor nerve. It is a striated muscle and arises from the orbital apex from the undersurface of the lesser wing of the sphenoid bone and courses anteriorly where it thins to a broad aponeurosis that inserts onto the anterior surface of the tarsal plate. In the lid of non-Asian persons, the supratarsal crease is created by the anterior extension of the levator into the pretarsal orbicularis oculi muscle and overlying skin. These aponeurotic fibers begin to send slips to the skin 2–3 mm above the superior margin of the tarsus. The levator aponeurosis then fans out to form medial and lateral horns that attach to the medial and lateral retinacula, respectively. The muscular portion is approximately 40 mm long, whereas the aponeurotic portion measures 15–20 mm.

During blepharoplasty, the integrity of the levator aponeurosis must be evaluated. Acquired ptosis of the upper eyelid often results from dehiscence of the levator from the tarsal plate. Additionally, overresection of the orbicularis muscle can inadvertently injure the aponeurosis.

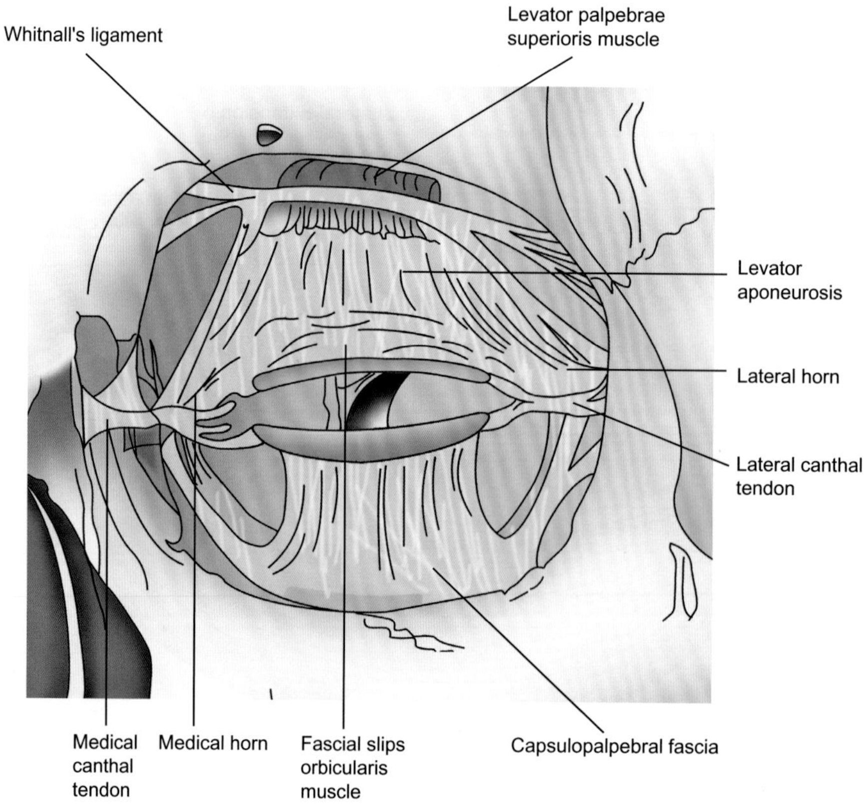

Figure 1-6. Eyelid retractors (left eye).

Deep to the levator lies Müller's muscle, a smooth muscle extension off the undersurface of the levator in the region of the aponeurotic-muscle junction (**Figure 1-1**). It is innervated by the sympathetic nervous system and travels inferiorly between the levator aponeurosis and conjunctiva, inserting into the superior margin of the tarsus. Fatty infiltration, as seen with aging, gives the muscle a yellowish color. Injury to the cervical sympathetic chain may results in Horner's syndrome with the triad of ptosis, miosis, and anhidrosis. Disruption of the sympathetic innervation to Müller's muscle typically results in about 2 mm of ptosis.

Lower Lid Retractors

The capsulopalpebral fascia is the lower eyelid equivalent of the levator aponeurosis (**Figure 1-6**). However, unlike the levator muscle, the fascia contains no muscle. The capsulopalpebral fascia envelops the inferior oblique muscle and then reunites as the inferior transverse ligament or Lockwood ligament (analogous to Whitnall's ligament in the upper eyelid) before passing anterosuperiorly onto the inferior border of the tarsus. The inferior rectus muscle acts as a lower lid retractor by transmitting its action to the capsulopalpebral fascia. When the capsulopalpebral fascia is dehiscent, entropion can occur.

Sympathetically innervated smooth muscle fibers are also found in the lower eyelid in the form of Horner's muscle—the inferior tarsal muscle (**Figure 1-1**). Horner's muscle does not insert directly onto the inferior tarsal border but rather into the fascia several millimeters below the tarsal border.

Conjuctiva

The conjunctiva is the mucous membrane covering of the eye. It covers the sclera and cornea, then reflects back to line the inner surface of the eyelids. It is firmly adherent to the overlying tarsal plates and the sympathetic tarsal muscle of Müller. The caruncle, a small mound of tissue, is found at the medial canthal angle. It consists of modified skin that contains fine hairs, sebaceous glands, and sweat glands.

Neurovascular Anatomy

Motor Nerves

The temporal and zygomatic branches of the facial nerve (CNVII) innervate the orbicularis oculi muscle (**Figure 1-7A**). The levator palpebra superioris is innervated by the superior branch of the oculomotor nerve (CNIII), whereas Müller's muscle and the inferior tarsal muscle rely on sympathetic innervation.

Sensory Nerves

Sensory innervation to the eyelids is supplied by branches of the trigeminal nerve (CNV) (**Figure 1-7B**). Terminal branches of the ophthalmic nerve (CNV_1)—supraorbital, supratrochlear, and

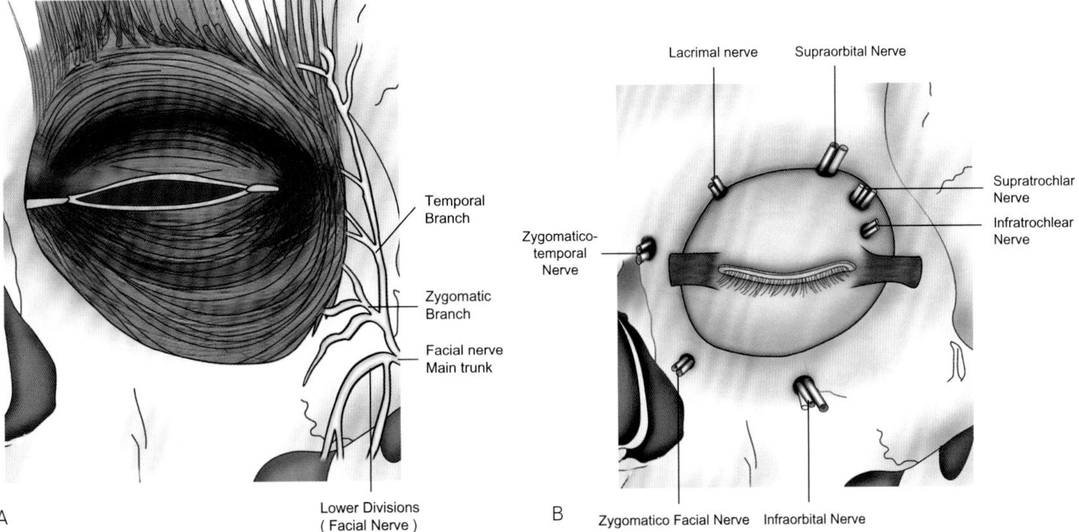

Figure 1-7. (A) Motor innervation to orbicularis oculi. (B) Sensory innervation to eyelids and periorbital region.

lacrimal—supply sensation to the upper eyelid and forehead. The infratrochlear nerve (branch of CNV_1) receives sensory information from the medial-most portion of both the upper and lower eyelids. Similarly, the zygomaticotemporal branch of the maxillary nerve (CNV_2) supplies the lateral portion of the upper eyelid and temple. The remainder of the sensory innervation to the lower lid is derived from branches of CNV_2. The infraorbital nerve supplies the central lower eyelid, whereas the zygomaticofacial nerve supplies the lateral portion of the lower eyelid.

Blood Supply and Lymphatics

The eyelids have an extensive and highly collateralized blood supply **(Figure 1-8)**. The posterior eyelid lamellae receive blood through a series of vascular arcades. In the upper lid, the arterial marginal arcade (**Figure 1-8A**) runs approximately 4 mm from the lid's free margin and a peripheral arcade extends along the superior border of the tarsus between the levator aponeurosis and Müller's muscle where it is at risk to injuring during blepharoptosis surgery. The arterial vascular arcades are supplied medially by the superior medial palpebral vessel (terminal branch of the ophthalmic artery) and laterally by the superior lateral palpebral vessel from the lacrimal artery.

Similar to the upper lid, the lower lid also has an arterial marginal arcade, which is about 2 mm from the lid margin. There is no well-defined peripheral arcade in the lower lid. The lower lid arcade receives its bloody supply from the medial and lateral inferior palpebral vessels.

The venous drainage system **(Figure 1-8B)** is organized similarly to the arterial system but, as in most parts of the body, it is not as consistent. The bulk of the drainage eventually finds its way into the vessels of the facial system. Lymphatic drainage from the lateral portion of the eyelids drain into preauricular and parotid nodes, whereas the drainage from the medial segment of the lids empties into submandibular nodes.

Related Anatomy

Lacrimal System

The lacrimal system plays a vital role in protecting the globe. Tears are secreted by the lacrimal gland which is located laterally in the preaponeurotic compartment of the upper lid **(Figure 1-9)**. The blinking action of the eyelid helps distribute the tear film evenly and propel the film medially to the medial canthus where they enter the lacrimal system via the upper and lower lid puncta—located approximately 5–7 mm lateral to the medial canthus. The superior and inferior canaliculus combine to form the common canaliculus before entering the lacrimal sac. The lacrimal sac lies within the lacrimal fossa, a bony groove in the nasal bone, and represents the dilated superior portion of the nasolacrimal duct and is about 15 mm long. The lacrimal sac empties into the nasolacrimal duct, which in turns opens into the inferior meatus at the valve of Hasner.

Retro-Orbicularis Oculi Fat Pad

The retro-orbicularis oculi fat pad (ROOF) is a layer of fibrofatty soft tissue deep to the orbicularis oculi muscle and superficial to both the orbital rim and septum **(Figure 1-10)**. It extends medially from the superior orbital nerve foramen/notch to a varying distance laterally over the lateral orbit. The ROOF is crescent shaped and, in cadaver studies, was found on average to be roughly two-thirds the transverse orbital dimension in width and one-third the vertical orbital dimension in height.

Although the ROOF is not anatomically part of the eyelid, its anatomy is relevant, as ROOF resection is increasingly being performed at the time of upper lid blepharoplasty to reduce thickness and heaviness over the lateral brow. Fullness due to ROOF can be distinguished from prominent preaponeurotic fat on physical examination, as gentle pressure on the globe will not accentuate ROOF fullness as it will with excess subseptal fat in the medial and central compartments. Care must be taken during ROOF resection to avoid injury to the superior orbital nerve medially and the lacrimal gland laterally. Furthermore, adequate hemostasis is of the utmost importance because the supraorbital vessels lie on the undersurface of the lateral orbicularis oculi muscle as it connects the angular and frontal vessels medially and the deep preauricular vessels laterally.

Suborbicularis Oculi Fat Pad

The suborbicularis oculi fat pad (SOOF) is the inferior orbital analog of the ROOF. The SOOF is a hockey puck–shaped collection of fat found below the orbicularis oculi muscle in the supraperiosteal plane at or just below the inferior orbital rim on the

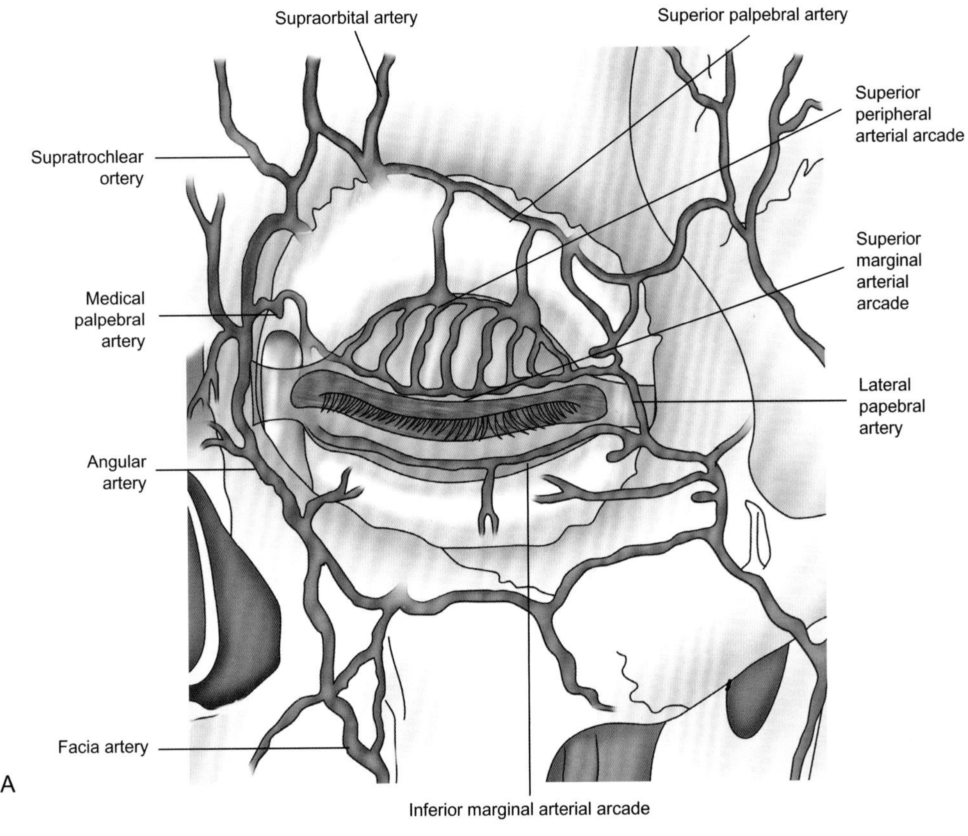

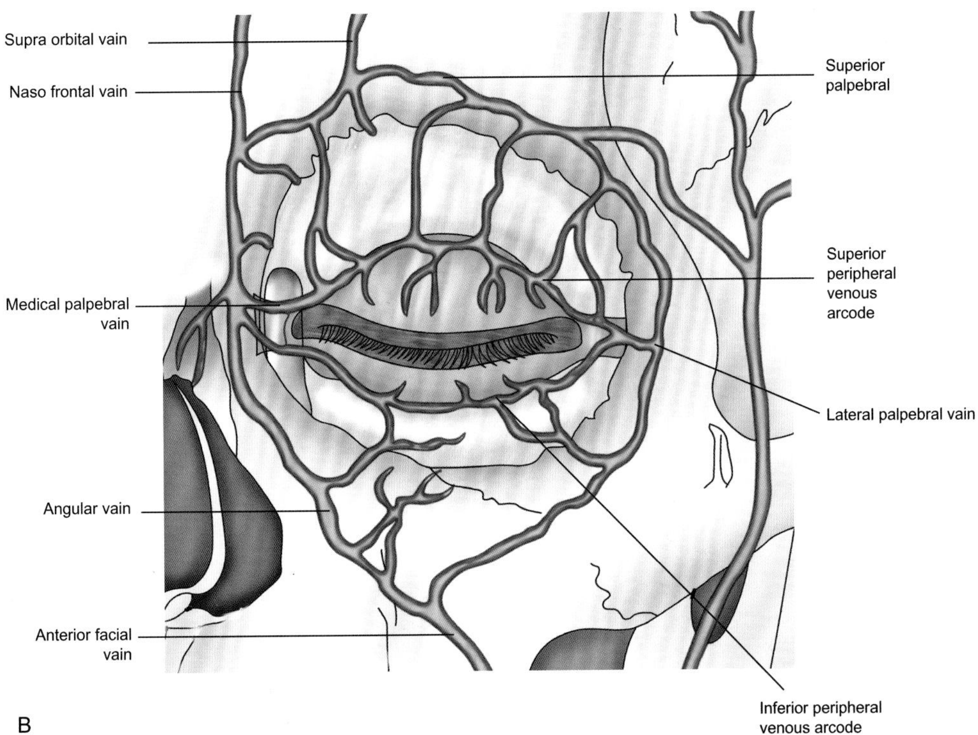

Figure 1-8. Arterial (A) and venous (B) blood supply to the eyelids (left eye).

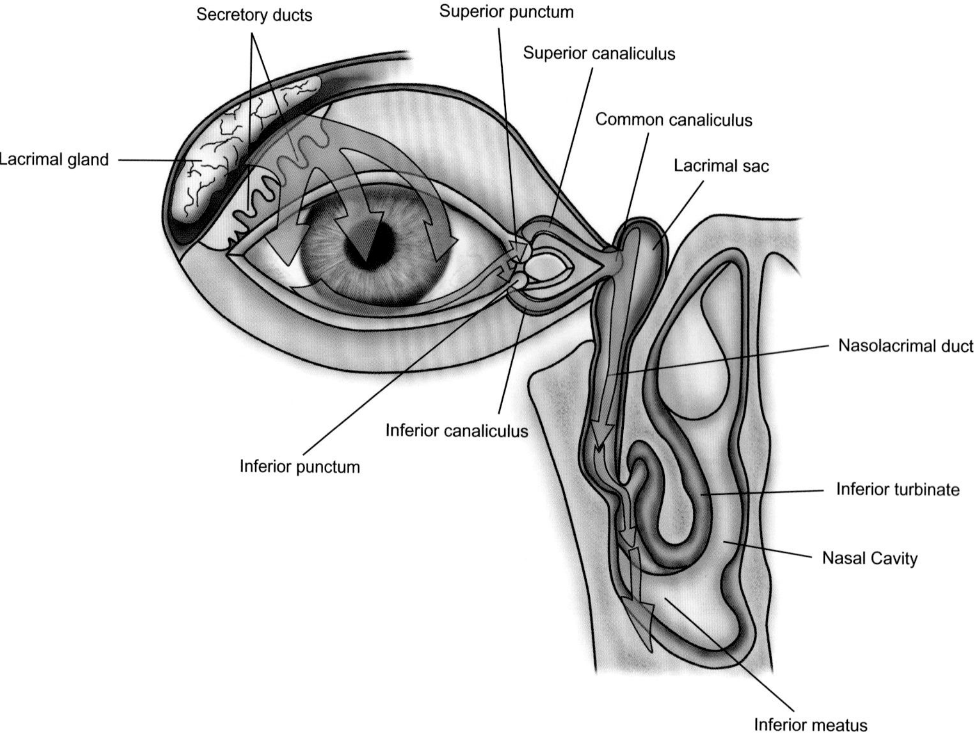

Figure 1-9. The lacrimal system. The direction of movement of the tear film is indicated by the arrows.

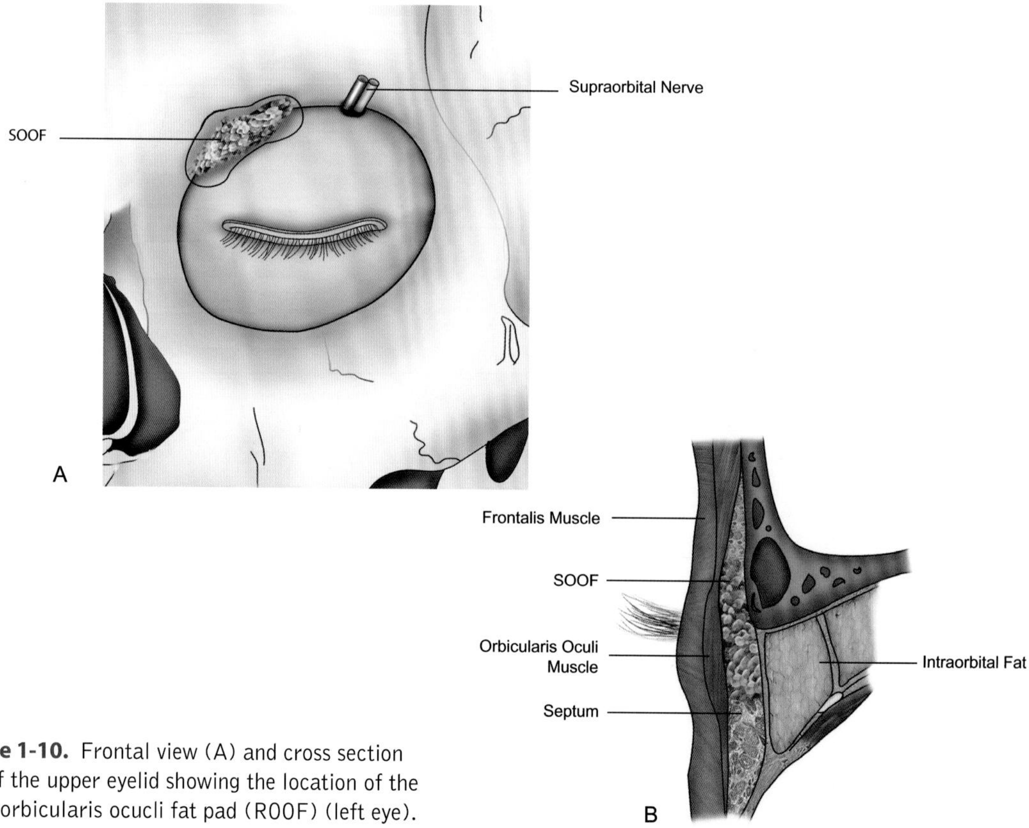

Figure 1-10. Frontal view (A) and cross section (B) of the upper eyelid showing the location of the retro-orbicularis ocucli fat pad (ROOF) (left eye).

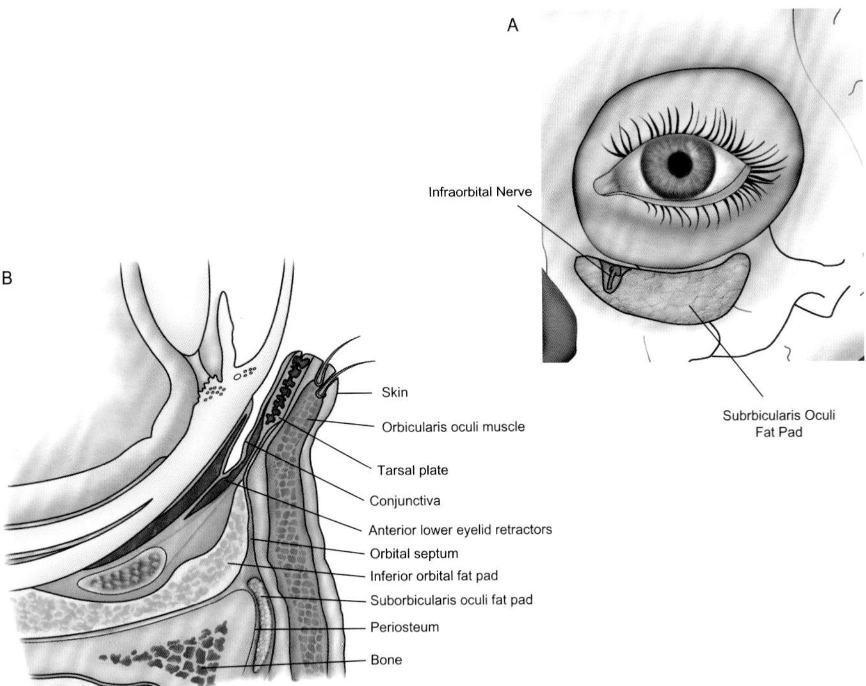

Figure 1-11. Frontal view (A) and cross section (B) of the lower eyelid showing the location of the suborbicularis oculi fat pad (SOOF) (Left eye).

zygoma (**Figure 1-11**). SOOF resection at the time of lower lid blepharoplasty is aimed at addressing prominence of the malar bags, the so called "jowls of the eye," caused by ptosis of the SOOF. Some methods of modern lower blepharoplasty seek to relocate the SOOF to correct for gravitational changes.

There are many causes of malar bags and include palpebral edema, subcutaneous skin excess, skin relaxation, and attenuation of the orbicularis oculi muscle. Worsening of malar bags with forward tilting of the head without change in the appearance of the malar bag with forceful eye closure is suggestive of malar bags caused by SOOF ptosis. Compared to ROOF resection, there are fewer critical structures in the infraorbital region; nevertheless, care must be taken during SOOF resection to avoid injury to the inferior orbital nerve, which may be within the medial aspect of the fat pad.

Asian Eyelid

Distinct anatomic differences distinguish the Asian eyelid from the Caucasian eyelid. The Asian eyelid displays more subcutaneous and suborbicularis fat and the preaponeurotic fat pad descends anterior to the tarsal plate resulting in a thickened or puffy appearing eyelid. Many people regard the Asian eyelid as a single eyelid—without a visible lid crease. However, three distinct morphologies can be seen: (1) single eyelid (no visible crease), (2) low eyelid crease (nasally tapered and low-seated), and (3) double eyelid (lid crease parallel to lid margin). The relative proportion of each morphology varies depending on the Asian race, but the majority do not have the double eyelid morphology.

When a supratarsal crease is present it is located only 6–7 mm above the lid margin as compared to 7–10 mm in most non-Asian persons. The absence of a supratarsal crease or a lower placement of the crease in the Asian upper eyelid is due to several factors: fusion of the orbital septum to the levator aponeurosis at a variable distance below the superior tarsal border, preaponeurotic fat pad protrusion and a thick subcutaneous fat layer preventing levator fibers from extending toward the skin near the superior tarsal border, and the primary insertion of the levator aponeurosis into the orbicularis muscle into the upper eyelid skin closer to the eyelid margin compared to Caucasians (**Figure 1-12**). Familiarity with the unique anatomy of the Asian eyelid is critical to the success of those surgeons performing blepharoplasty or lid explorations in patients of Asian descent.

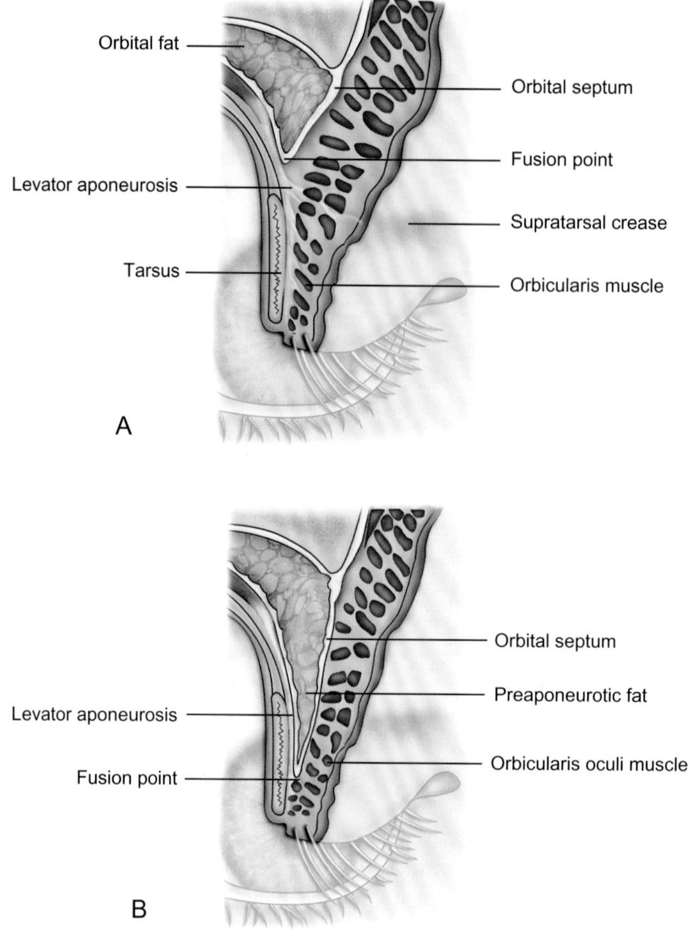

Figure 1-12. (A) Eyelid of a non-Asian person compared to (B) the eyelid of a person of Asian descent with the single eyelid morphology (no supratarsal crease).

Suggested Readings

1. Aiache AE, Ramirez OH. The suborbicularis oculi fat pads: An anatomic and clinical study. *Plast Reconstr Surg* 1995; 95(1):37–42.
2. Bilyk JR. Periocular and orbital anatomy. *Curr Open Ophthalmula* 1995; 6(5):53–58.
3. Dioxanes MT, Anderson RL. Oriental eyelids. An anatomic study. *Arch Ophthalmol* 1984;102(8):1232–1235.
4. Dutton JJ. Clinical anatomy of the eyelids. In: Yanoff M, Duker J, eds. Ophthalmology. 2nd ed. St. Louis, MO: Mosby, 2003.
5. Gausas RE. Advances in applied anatomy of the eyelid and orbit. *Curr Opin Ophthalmol* 2004;15(5): 422–425.
6. Jeong S, Lemke BN, Dortzbach RK et al. The Asian upper eyelid: An anatomical study with comparison to the Caucasian eyelid. *Arch Ophthalmol* 1999; 117(7):907–912.
7. Kontis TC, Papel ID, Larrabee WF. Surgical anatomy of the eyelids. *Facial Plast Surg* 1994;10(1):5.
8. May JW, Jr., Fearon J, Zingarelli P. Retro-orbicularis oculus fat (ROOF) resection in aesthetic blepharoplasty: A 6-year study in 63 patients. *Plast Reconstr Surg* 1990;86(4):682–689.
9. Oh CS, Chung IH, Kim YS et al. Anatomic variations of the infraorbital fat compartment. *J Plast Reconstr Aesthet Surg* 2006;59(4):376–379.
10. Persichetti P, Di Lella F, Delfino S et al. Adipose compartments of the upper eyelid: Anatomy applied to blepharoplasty. *Plast Reconstr Surg* 2004;113(1): 373–378.
11. Riordan-Eva P. Anatomy and embryology of the eyes. In: Riordan-Eva P, Whitcher JP, eds. Vaughan & Asbury's General Ophthalmology. New York: McGraw-Hill, 2003.

2

Aesthetic Evaluation of the Periorbital Region

Kofi Boahene, MD

The eyes are the primary focus of most social interactions and account for a large part of the expressiveness of the face. Contour changes around the eyes are among the earliest signs of facial aging. Aging changes in the periorbital region are not easily concealed and are common reasons why patients first seek aesthetic consultations. Periorbital rejuvenation can brighten one's overall appearance and restore confidence. A comprehensive aesthetic analysis of the periorbital region based on the anatomic changes in the brow, eyelid skin, muscles, orbital fat, and cheeks should form the basis of all rejuvenation procedures.

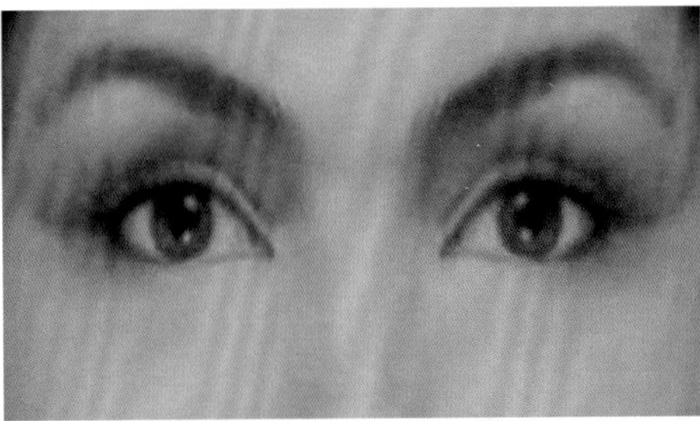

Figure 2-1. The eyelid in youth. In youth, the upper eyelid transitions smoothly from the brow to the lid margin without much interruption. The lid crease is low with only 2–3 mm pretarsal skin showing. Note the brow-to-crease distance. The lower lid blends into the cheek without revealing the orbital rim, fat compartments, or malar septum.

The Periorbital Region in Youth

The goal of aesthetic periorbital rejuvenation is to restore a youthful and rested appearance. In youth, the upper eyelid transition smoothly from the eyebrow without a deep supraorbital sulcus (**Figure 2-1**). The eyelids are full and not hollow. The skin is crisp with no wrinkles and has good elastic recoil. The supratarsal crease is low with only 2–3 mm pretarsal skin showing. The upper eyelid margin sits about 1 mm just inferior to the upper limbus and makes a gentle arch with a peak just nasal to the central pupil. The upper eyelids are framed by the eyebrows, which in females sit just above the superior orbital rim, and in males at the orbital rim. A lot has been written about the shape of the eyebrow and where the ideal peak should reside. Considered on an individual basis, however, one will find that the often described ideal brow aesthetic features is not universal and depends or several factors including the shape of the face, intercanthal distance, and ethnicity. In fact, the standards of an attractive brow changes with time reflecting contemporary fashion and culture of the time. In the 1940s and 1950s, female movie stars often removed their eyebrows completely. Then in the 1960s, the bushy brow was in vogue. In the 1980s eyebrows thinned again, but presently thick eyebrows are back in style. Determining and restoring the youthful brow shape on a given patient rather than using a predetermine ideal will often result in a balanced look following periorbital rejuvenation. It is helpful to review pictures of patients in their youth to gain an understanding of their aging process.

In youth, the lower eyelid margin sits just above the inferior limbus and is well apposed to the globe and has good recoil on a snap test. The lowest point of the lid margin is just temporal to the central pupil. An inferior tarsal crease is found 5–6 mm below the ciliary margin and corresponds to the transition from pretarsal to preseptal orbicularis oculi muscle. There is a smooth transition to the malar region without significant contour breaks at the orbital rim (**Figure 2-1**).

General Evaluation of Patients Seeking Aesthetic Periorbital Rejuvenation

As with all cosmetic procedures, successful outcome depends on selecting patients properly, correctly identifying their specific concerns, and establishing achievable goals. The patient's motivation should be determined prior to aesthetic rejuvenation. Recent relationship changes may hint at patients who are seeking aesthetic enhancement to fill an inner void and will not be satisfied by surgery. On the contrary, individuals who have considered rejuvenation options for awhile, want to look more awake, or want to look their best for a new job are usually happy after surgery. The patient should be medically and psychologically sound to undergo the procedure as well as the recovery process. The postoperative period in eyelid surgery may be depressing for some individuals especially when they are bruised and swollen. Patients who already have a history of depression and are not optimally treated with antidepressants or lack an appropriate support system may become worse after surgery. Medical conditions such as thyroid disease and other inflammatory eye diseases that may cause premature periorbital aging should always be sought and appropriately addressed. A history of bleeding disorder, dry eye syndrome, glaucoma, and myasthenia gravis should be determined. A medication list should be obtained and should include nonprescription and herbal supplements. Schirmer's test is important when dry eye is suspected. This may be performed by first applying topical ophthalmic anesthetic drops, then applying a Schirmer strip and taking measurements at 5-minute intervals. If there is less than 5 mm travel of moisture in 5 minutes, corneal dryness may be a problem and warrants further investigation. Individuals with a questionable ophthalmic history should be comprehensively evaluated by an ophthalmologist.

Assessing for Dynamic Changes around the Eye

Periorbital analysis should include assessment of dynamic changes around the eye during facial animation. The presence of deep creases in the lateral orbital region (crow's feet) glabella, and nasal root upon facial animation may eventually lead to undesirable static wrinkles (**Figure 2-2**). Prophylactic treatment with botulinum toxin may be considered. The function of the orbital muscles should be recorded. Establishing the presence of Bell's phenomenon is particularly essential. This is done by instructing the patient to close their eyes and then attempting to forcibly open their closed eyes. If Bell's phenomenon is intact, the globes will be directed upward and inward by the pull of the superior rectus muscle. With an intact Bell's phenomenon, the globe will be protected during sleep and will better tolerate some degree of postoperative lagophthalmus. Intact function of the ocular muscles as well as the levator should be determined.

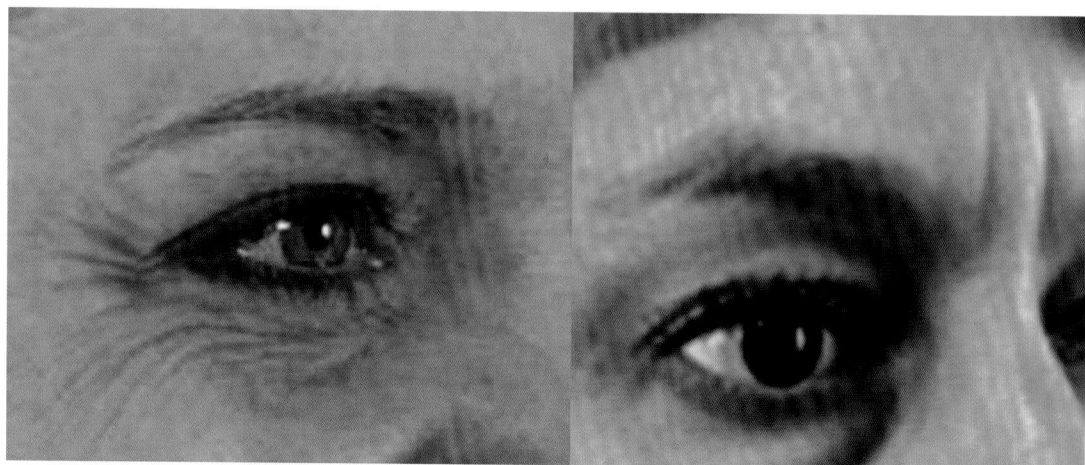

Figure 2-2. Dynamic periorbital wrinkles.

Analysis of the Upper Eyelid

Analysis of the upper lid may begin with evaluating the position of the eyelid margin. Ptosis of the upper eyelid is diagnosed when the lid margin sits more than 1 mm below the upper limbus. In severe Ptosis where lid margin is 4 mm or more below the upper limbus, approximately 50% of the visual field may be blocked. While severe ptosis is easily recognized, mild ptosis (1-2 mm) require attentive evaluation otherwise they are easily missed **(Figure 2-3)**. When ptosis is diagnosed, a determination should be made whether this is true ptosis resulting from levator palpebral muscle pathology, inadequate sympathetic input to Mueller's muscle or pseudoptosis from the upper lid being weighted down by a prolapsed brow. When levator palpebral aponeurosis is attenuated as a result of aging, the supratarsal crease is higher than usual or may be completely lost. In such cases, lowering the supratarsal crease with levator advancement is essential.

The upper lid skin should be evaluated for pigmentary changes and skin tags. These surface changes may be congenital or may herald a systemic problem that warrants further medical evaluation. The presence of xanthelesma, for example, may be associated with elevated serum lipids requiring treatment with medications.

Next, the upper lid skin should be analyzed for wrinkles or laxity. There is a fundamental difference between the management of the two, as laxity is not the same as wrinkling **(Figure 2-4)**. Laxity of the upper eyelid skin is a result of lost elasticity with stretching and sagging over time. Wrinkling is caused by loss of dermal collagen and subcutaneous fat as a result of aging and photodamage. Elongated and lax lid skin requires conservative trimming for tightening, whereas wrinkles are best treated with resurfacing either with laser or chemical peel. The two approaches are not interchangeable and will not achieve equivalent results.

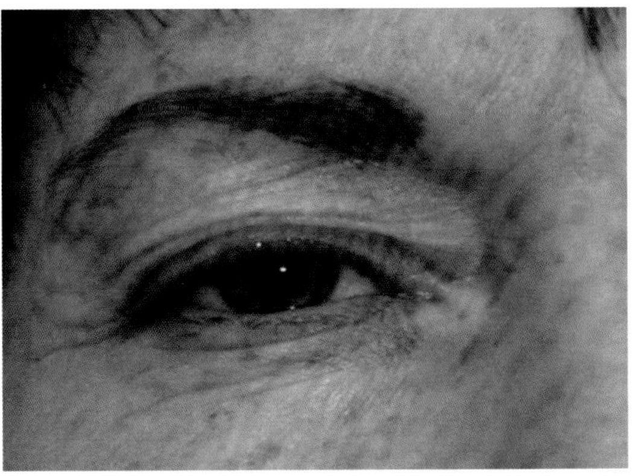

Figure 2-3. Upper eyelid ptosis. At primary gaze, the upper lid margin is seen 1 mm above the papillary reflex which reflects severe ptosis. Although severe ptosis is easily noted, identifying milder forms requires attentive analysis.

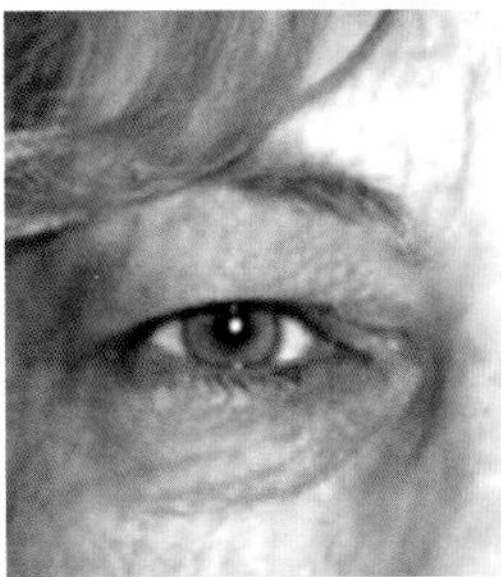
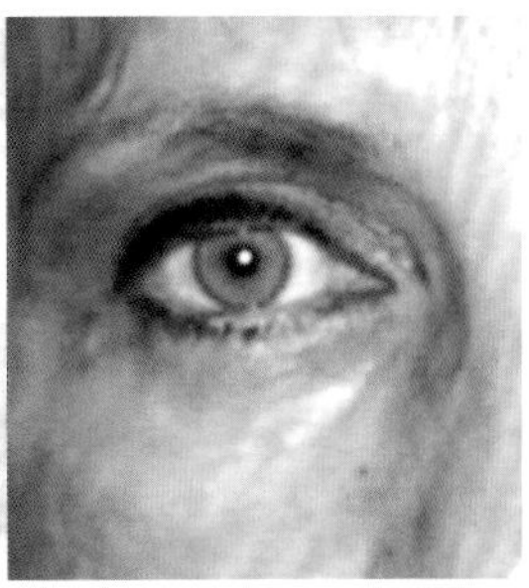

Figure 2-4. Eyelid wrinkles should be distinguished from eyelid laxity. Wrinkles respond to resurfacing with either laser or chemical peeling (right).

Assessing laxity of the upper eyelid skin should always be done in conjunction with determining the adequacy of orbital volume. Loss and shifting of orbital fat, and volume, is commonly seen with aging. If the eyelids are already short on volume, there is no good reason to add to the deficiency by excisional blepharoplasty. With loss of volume, the upper eyelid becomes deflated and appears saggy. This may first appear as be a small roll of upper eyelid skin that often invites excision. Excising this apparent upper lid excess will result in more volume loss with further hollowing. Inadequate orbital fat volume maybe determined by manually elevating the brow. With the brow elevated, a supraorbital hollow may be unmasked **(Figure 2-5)**. A mild degree of hollowness may be hereditary and was usually present when the patient was younger. Such patients may also have naturally low eyebrows. Caution should be exercised in any volume-reducing procedures in such individuals. Asking the patient to look down

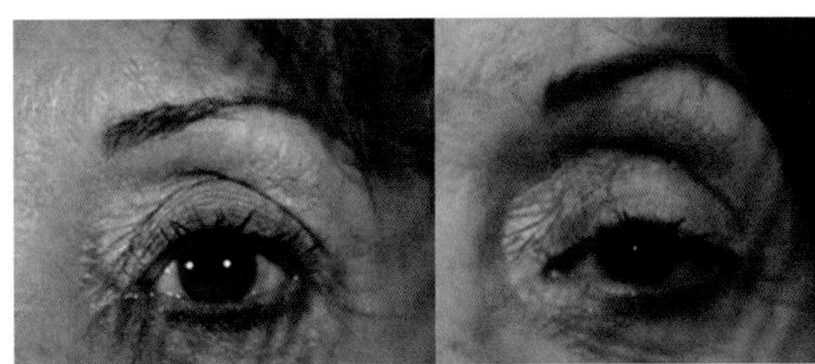

Figure 2-5. Signs of upper eyelid deflation (left) becomes accentuated following brow elevation (right) revealing deep a supraorbital hollow.

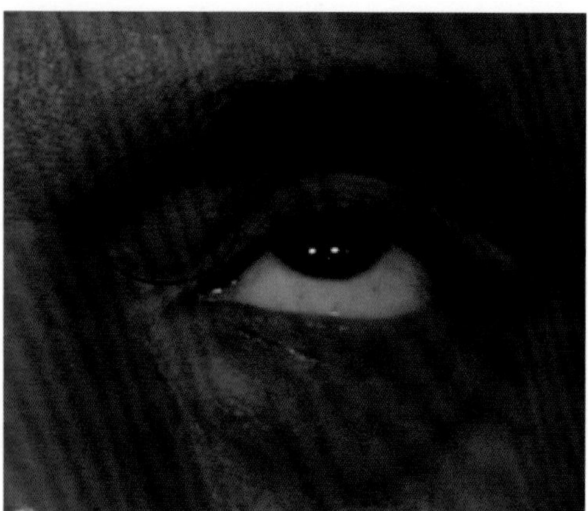

Figure 2-6. Medial upper eyelid bulge.

also helps is determining adequacy of upper eyelid volume.

Fullness in the upper eyelid should also be analyzed for volume shifts and other potential causes. It is common to see bulging of the medial fat pad (**Figure 2-6**). This is best treated by direct fat resection. Medial upper lid fat bulging that occurs as an isolated finding may be addressed via a transconjuctival approach. Lateral upper eyelid fullness from fat shifting is rare and should raise suspicion for a tumor or a prolapsing lacrimal gland that may require resuspension. Lateral upper eyelid fullness resulting from eyebrow ptosis is a distinct problem that should be corrected with a temporal brow procedure rather than an eyelid procedure.

The position of the upper eyelid crease is an essential feature that reflects youth. As noted, in youth the eyelid crease is low and reveals only 2–3 mm of pretarsal skin. Individuals seeking periorbital rejuvenation often have the position of the eyelid crease obscured by the appearance of redundant skin or fold. It is important to manually elevate the skin to reveal the position of the crease, which may be found to be too high and sometimes asymmetric. Lowering the eyelid crease with deliberate lower (6–9 mm) placement of incisions may be necessary to restore youthful appearance. Here, again, it is prudent look at pictures of patients in their youth to gain a sense of their individual lid aesthetics.

Analysis of the Eyebrow

The position, shape, and symmetry of the eyebrows are essential in eye beauty. The eyebrows are analogous to a picture frame: they should outline the eyes nicely but should not distract attention from the eyes. A heavy, drooped, misshapen, overly thin or excessively busy eyebrow can be distracting. The eyebrow position is determined by the balance between the major brow elevator (frontalis muscle) and depressors (lateral and medial portions of the orbicularis oculi muscles). The eyebrow is also supported by a foundation of subcutaneous and orbital fat much like how a foundation holds up a building. The ideal brow position should be determined on an individual basis but in general is above the superior orbital rim for females and at the rim for males. It is useful to review youthful pictures of the patient to get a sense of their ideal brow position. When a person's brows sit naturally low, this is often because there is not much natural fat present to prop them up. Excising what little fat there is may drop the brow even further as it collapses into the void. On the other hand, elevating naturally low eyebrows may unmask a hollow eye. One evidence of eyebrow ptosis is the presences of deep forehead rhytids. Patients with drooping eyebrows reflexively elevated their brows with their frontalis muscle. Besides the wrinkles that ensue, patients may complain of a lower brow position during the latter half of the day. Botulinum toxin injected to improve forehead creases in such patients may worsen their brow ptosis. When considering brow ptosis, the position of the medial and the temporal brow should be assessed independently. Often, correction of the temporal brow position alone may be all that is needed, whereas elevating the medial brow shows signs of overdone surgery. Volume depletion in the lateral brow and periorbital region will result in lost of the lateral brow foundation and subsequent brow descent. In such cases, volume replacement may be the best approach to correction. The natural eyebrow peak should also be determined on an individual basis. In females, the eyebrow peaks somewhere between the lateral limbus and the lateral canthus. Women seeking periorbital rejuvenation have often shaved or plucked their eyebrows to achieve a desirable brow contour. This practice should be determined, as it can often blur correct analysis of brow contour and position.

The relationship between the eyebrow and the upper eyelid is essential in restoring a youthful appearance. There is quite a distance between the upper eyelid crease and the eyebrow margin in youth. This distance is shortened by lateral hooding and brow descent. The need for lateral browpexy or volume restoration should be determined when considering upper eyelid procedures to improve or maintain the brow to upper crease distance.

Analysis of the Lower Eyelid

Aesthetic analysis of the lower lid should include evaluation of the status of the supporting ligaments, shape and position of the lid margin, and the contour changes in the lower eyelid and lid–cheek interface. With aging, the canthal ligaments become lax and rounding of the eyelid margin and increased scleral show occurs as a result. The integrity of the canthal ligaments can be assessed by gentle outward distraction or inferior retraction. Too much lid distraction and slow recoil suggests laxity of the canthal ligaments. Canthopexy should be considered when canthal laxity is identified. The size, shape, and symmetry of the lateral scleral triangle should be noted. Rounding of the lateral scleral triangle is a telltale sign of canthal laxity of previous lower eyelid surgery and must be avoided or corrected by appropriately addressing the lateral canthal support system.

A common aesthetic complain about the lower eyelids is the presence of dark circles. Dark circles around the lower eyelid may be the result of congenital dermal melanocytosis, postinflammatory hyperpigmentation, eyelid skin laxity/redundancy, chronic inflammation, or hypervascularity seen deep to the skin. Dermal melanocytosis and postinflammatory hyperpigmentation may respond to bleach agents and superficial peeling. Dark circle resulting from eyelid contour changes because of bulging or hollowing respond well to surgical correction or filler contouring. Dark circles that are a result of lower-lid hypervascularity are difficult to treat. Eyelid bleaching is usually not effective and resurfacing procedures may exacerbate the appearance of the hypervascularity, as the lid becomes thinner and more translucent from pigment loss.

Superficial skin changes in the lower eyelid should then be determined. As in the upper eyelid, fine wrinkles should be distinguished from dynamic wrinkles and skin laxity. Contour changes in the lower eyelid and the eyelid–cheek junction may be considered as regions of bulges (volume gain) or depressions (volume loss).The anatomic correlate to these bulges and depressions should be determined and should form the basis of aesthetic correction (**Figure 2-7**). Lower eyelid bulges can stem from prolapsed orbital fat, prominent orbicularis oculi muscle, lax skin, and edematous eyelid. Around the malar region and the eyelid–cheek junction, depressions can be seen along the orbital rim, tear trough region, and malar septum. A triangular malar bulge is often seen adjacent to a malar septal depression. The orbital fat may prolapse as the fibrous septa composing the orbital support and suspensory system weakens with age. Prolapsed orbital fat can often be distinguished into medial, central, and lateral components each with a characteristic shape (**Figure 2-7**). Bulging of the lower eyelid resulting from chronic edema can be distinguished from orbital fat prolase by the lack of compartmentalization in the former. Bulges from prominent orbicularis oculi muscle are usually seen along the lid margin and become more prominent during a smile. These can be seen in youth and may not necessarily need correction. The areas of periorbital depression usually correspond anatomically to regions of deep septodermal attachment (**Figure 2-7**). The depression along the orbital rim results from the attachment of the orbitomalar ligament and is accentuated by bulging orbital fat above and prolapsing suborbicularis oculi fat and cheek fat below. The outline of the depression along the orbital rim is often triangular in shape with its medial half representing the tear trough hollow described by flowers. Anatomically, the malar depression corresponds to the malar septum or the orbitozygomatic ligaments. This depression can become more prominent as the triangular malar mound bulges up. Along the lower eyelid proper, the deep attachment at the confluence between the tarsus, orbital septum and the lower eyelid retractor creates a depression that may become pronounced by a prominent roll of the pretarsal orbicularis oculi muscle above and bulging orbital fat below. A combination of techniques targeting the various bulges and depression in the lower lid and cheek is often necessary to restore the youthful lower eyelid.

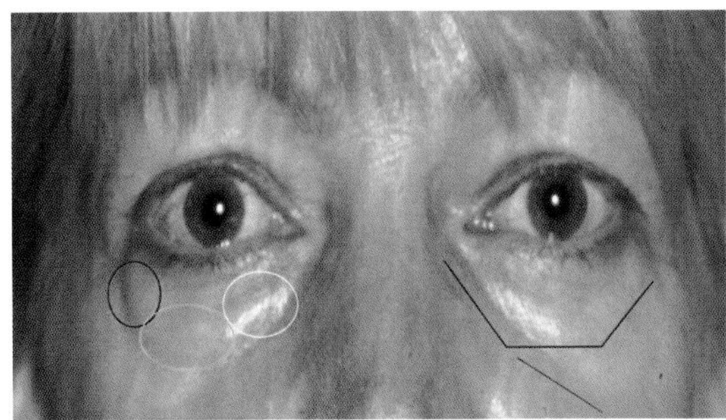

Figure 2-7. Bulges and depression of the lower eyelid and cheek. Contour changes in the lower eyelid–cheek complex may be seen as a result of volume shifts with areas of gain showing bulges (colored circles) and areas of loss showing depressions (colored lines). Lines of depression are seen coinciding with regions of deep dermal retaining ligaments: orbital rim ligament and malar septal ligament.

The Positive and Negative Vector Globe–Orbital Relationship

The relationship of the anterior globe to the orbital rim, orbital fat, and cheek mass should be examined. An orbit that shows retrusion of the inferior orbital rim relative to the cornea has been described as a negative vector orbit. A positive vector orbit has the inferior orbital rim relatively anterior to the globe. The negative vector orbit exhibits eye proptosis, fat herniation, deep nasojugal groove, and recession of cheek mass. With aging, both the orbital skeletal platform and soft tissue are believed to involute. In this manner, the aging orbit may increasingly display negative vector features such as scleral show, prominent medial orbital fat, and deep nasojugal folds. These features have been found to be related to an increased dissatisfaction in standard lower blepharoplasty where fat excision accentuates orbital proptosis and may result in lid retraction.

Photo Documentation

Proper photo documentation is essential for reviewing details that may have been missed during the initial evaluation. Twelve standard photographic views are necessary for a comprehensive documentation of the preorbital region.

- Full face frontal
- Full face oblique views
- Close-up frontal eyes open
- Close-up lateral views, eyes open
- Close-up frontal upgaze
- Close-up lateral views, upgaze
- Close-up frontal eyes closed
- Close-up lateral views, eyes closed

Summary

Aesthetic analysis of the eyelids should be anatomic based and systematic to identify correctible aging changes. Restoration of youth rather than transformation should be the goal of eyelid rejuvenation and thus reviewing youthful pictures are helpful. Identifying high-risk features such as the negative vector eye, hollow eyes, and weak supporting canthal ligament should be a priority. Aesthetic periorbital analysis should be sensitive to contour changes resulting from volume shifts and depletion. When approached in this manner, periorbital rejuvenation can produce youthful results that are natural and long lasting.

Suggested Readings

1. Ellenbogen, R. Transcoronal eyebrow lift with concomitant upper blepharoplasty. Plast. Reconstr. *Surg.* 1983;71:490.
2. Angres, G. G. Blepharopigmentation and eyebrow enhancement techniques for maximum cosmetic results. Ann. *Ophthalmol.* 1985;17:605.
3. Fagien, S. Advanced rejuvenative upper blepharoplasty: Enhancing aesthetics of the upper periorbita. Plast. Reconstr. *Surg.* 2000;110:278–291
4. Fagien, S. Algorithm for canthoplasty: The lateral retinacular suspension: A simplified suture canthopexy. Plast. Reconstr. *Surg.* 1999;103:2042.
5. Epstein JS. Management of infraorbital dark circles. A significant cosmetic concern. *Arch Facial Plast Surg.* 1999;1:303–307.
6. Lowe NJ, Wieder JM, Shorr N et al. Infraorbital pigmented skin: Preliminary observations of laser therapy. Dermatol. *Surg.* 1995;21:767–770.
7. Goldberg RA, McCann JD, Fiaschetti D, Ben Simon GJ. What causes eyelid bags? Analysis of 114 consecutive patients. Plast. Reconstr. *Surg.* 2005;15;115(5):1395–1402; discussion 1403–1404.
8. Flowers RS. Tear trough implants for correction of tear trough deformities. Clin. Plast. Surg. 1993; 20:403.
9. Jelks GW, Jelks EB. Preoperative evaluation of the blepharoplasty patient. Bypassing the pitfalls. Clin. Plast. *Surg.* 1993;20:213.
10. Pessa JE, Desvigne LD, Lambros VS, Nimerick J, Sugunan B, Zadoo VP. Changes in ocular globe-to-orbital rim position with age: Implications for aesthetic blepharoplasty of the lower eyelids. Aesthet. Plast. *Surg.* 1999;23(5):337–42.
11. Elder, H. Importance of fat conservation in lower blepharoplasy. Aesthet. Plast. *Surg.* 1997;21:168.

3

Upper Eyelid Blepharoplasty

Lisa A. Earnest, MD and Ira D. Papel, MD

Introduction

The eyes play a central role in facial identity and expression and contribute significantly to the overall appearance of the face. There is great diversity in eye color and shape within and between different ethnic groups. Unfortunately, the eyes are one of the first areas of the face to demonstrate aging changes as a result of gravity and photodamage.

Aging changes in the periorbital region typically become apparent in individuals in their third decade of life. These changes may first manifest as "crow's feet", or "smile lines" arising from the lateral canthal region and progress to excess skin and fat pseudoherniation present in the substance of the upper eyelid. The overlying, lax skin and bulging fat, along with eyebrow ptosis, contribute to the appearance of a "tired" look. Patients begin to feel that their external appearance does not adequately reflect how they feel inside.

Upper blepharoplasty is a commonly performed procedure to address the aging changes of the upper eyelid. The procedure typically includes the excision of excess skin from the upper eyelid and removal of pseudoherniating fat as appropriate. It may be performed in conjunction with other facial rejuvenation procedures such as brow lift or lower blepharoplasty or alone, depending on the needs and desires of the patient.

Facial Analysis

Because the position of the eyebrows impacts the overall appearance of the eyes the analysis should begin with consideration of eyebrow position. The ideal brow position for a female is just above the superior orbital rim centrally and laterally. A brow elevation procedure should be considered in cases where the brow position is lower than ideal. Removal of excess eyelid skin when the brow is low may exacerbate brow ptosis.

The position of the brow should be evaluated when the patient is animated and when in repose. Patients with a low brow may habitually contract the brow elevators to keep the brows lifted above the orbital rim. In these cases, deep forehead rhytids will be present. In order to assess the true brow position, ask the patient to close their eyes for several seconds to relax the brow. Evaluate the position immediately after eye opening when the brow elevators are relaxed (**Figure 3-1**).

Eyelid evaluation consists of examining for excess skin and fat pseudoherniation in the medial and central compartments. Patients with very heavy lateral brows may require fat removal from beneath the orbicularis muscle near the lateral brow to relieve the weighted look of the heavy lateral brow. The upper lid should overlie the superior limbus in a position just above the pupil. The average palpebral opening is 10–12 mm high and 28–30 mm wide. Evaluation for palpebral fissure symmetry is essential to identify preexisting eyelid ptosis that will become more noticeable after eyelid surgery. The eyelid crease should be deep in the Caucasian female and lie in a position 9–10 mm above the lash line. This crease in the male should be shallower and lie in a position 8 mm above the lash line.

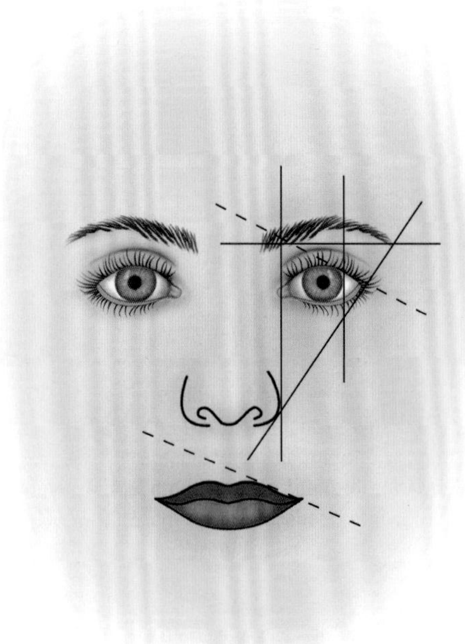

Figure 3-1. Brow and eyelid aesthetic ideals.

Preoperative Considerations

Preoperative blepharoplasty evaluation must include an inquiry into a history of dry eyes, prior eyelid surgery, or recent Botox use. The presence of ptosis must be documented and is best done so with documentation of the margin-to-reflex distance-1 (MRD_1), the distance from the central papillary light reflex to the upper lid margin. Patients with minimal ptosis (2 mm or less) may undergo a phenylephrine eyedrop test to determine the function of Müller's muscle in the ptotic eye and to unmask a possible ptosis in the opposite eye. If the MRD_1 increases by at least 1.5 mm, Müller's muscle may be considered functional and the patient a candidate for ptosis repair with Müller's muscle conjunctival resection. To check the contralateral eye for ptosis, the treated eye is covered and the contralateral eye checked for subsequent decrease in the MRD_1 by 1.5 mm. When present, this is an illustration of Herring's law (**Figure 3-2**).

For patients with thyroid eye disease, 6–12 months of disease stability is recommended prior to proceeding with upper blepharoplasty. For patients who have undergone recent Lasik eye surgery, the ophthalmologic surgeon should be consulted to recommend a safe waiting period prior before proceeding with cosmetic blepharoplasty. The type of anesthesia the patient would prefer to undergo must be addressed preoperatively. Although the procedure is commonly performed with local anesthesia and intravenous sedation, some patients may feel more comfortable with general anesthesia or local anesthesia alone. The risks to the procedure, including scar, change in vision, and lagophthalmos should be stressed to the patient during the attainment of informed consent.

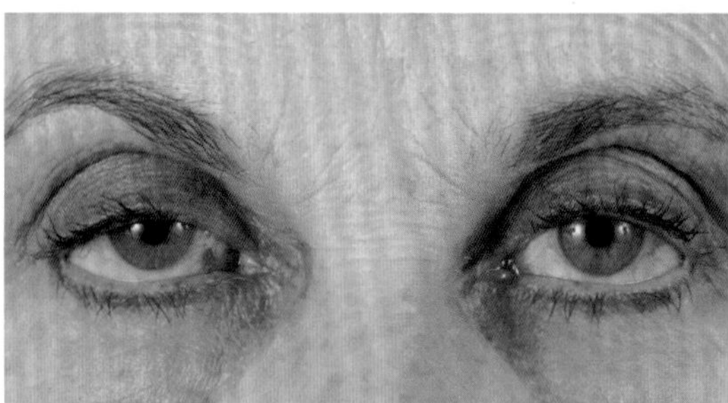

Figure 3-2. Demonstration of right upper eyelid ptosis.

Technique

Preoperative marking for incision and planned skin excision is one of the most important components of the procedure. The patient should first be evaluated in the upright position to assess skin overlap and the position of the lateral supratarsal crease. Only in cases of extensive lateral skin overhang beyond the lateral orbital rim will the incision need to extend beyond the lateral orbital rim. Staying within the supratarsal crease will contribute to scar camouflage. The medial extent of the incision should not extend beyond the naso-orbital depression onto the nasal skin as this may result in webbing. The remainder of the incision marking can be performed in the operating room with the patient in the supine position. With the lower incision located within the supratarsal crease, the upper incision is designed using forceps to pinch the excess skin (**Figure 3-3**).

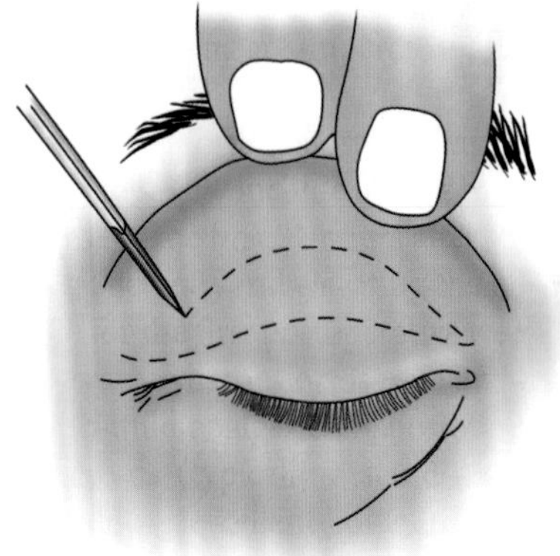

Figure 3-3. Eyelid markings for upper blepharoplasty.

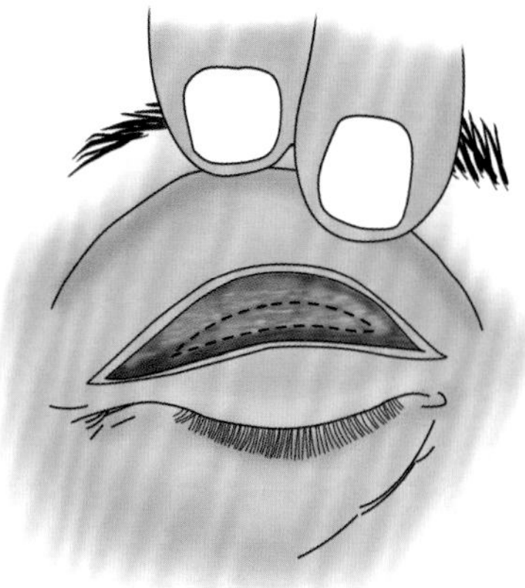

Figure 3-4. Excision of skin.

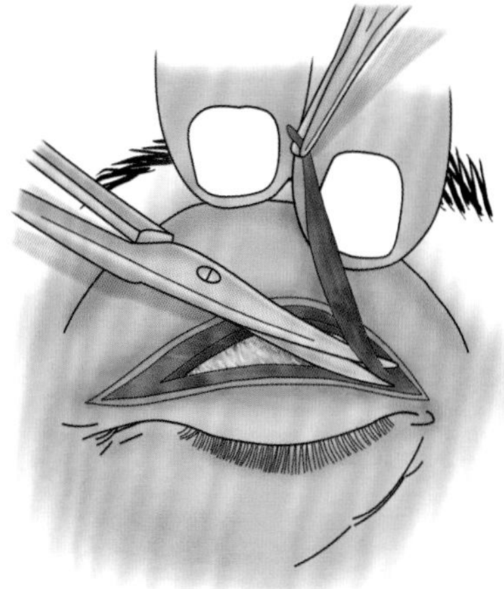

Figure 3-5. Excision of orbicularis muscle strip.

Once marking is completed, the skin is injected with 1 % lidocaine with 1:100,000 epinephrine in a volume of 1.0–2.0 mL, and the face is prepped and draped. The skin incision is performed with a #15 blade and the skin elevated with a pair of small dissecting scissors (**Figure 3-4**).

A strip of orbicularis oculi muscle is then resected just above the inferior incision using small dissecting scissors (**Figure 3-5**).

Once the skin and muscle are excised, a small bipolar cautery is used to achieve hemostasis of the small preseptal vessels. If fat pseudoherniation was noted preoperatively, the preaponeurotic fat compartment should be gently teased out after dissection through the orbital septum (**Figure 3-6**).

This portion of the procedure is frequently more painful when addressing the nasal fat pad and may require injection of additional local anesthesia into the preaponeurotic space. Prior to transecting the

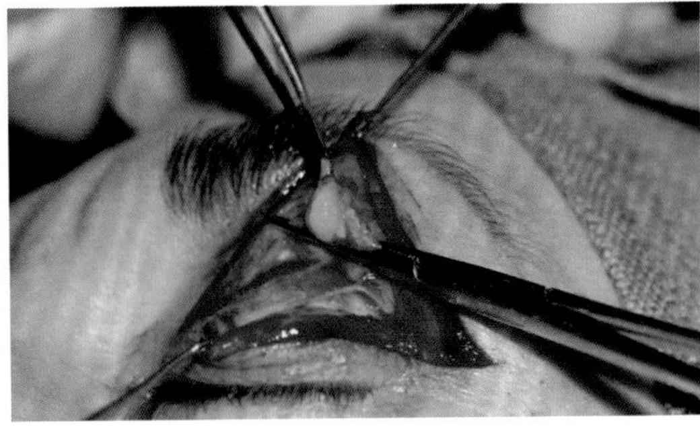

Figure 3-6. Preaponeurotic fat excision.

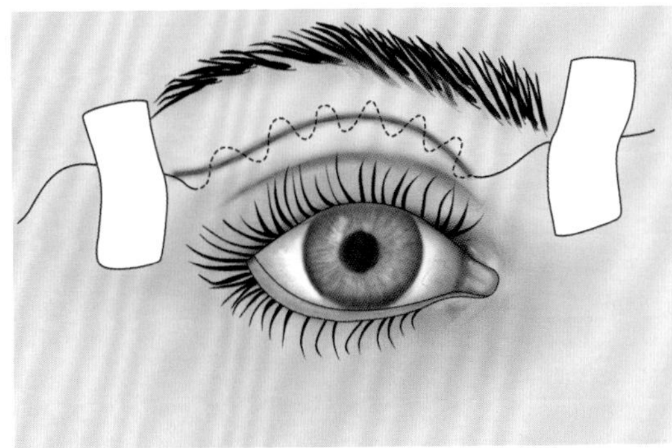

Figure 3-7. Closure of incision.

fat, the stalk is cauterized with a bipolar cautery to avoid bleeding. The wound is closed with running or interrupted sutures of 6-0 polypropylene and possibly interspersed 6-0 fast-absorbing plain gut depending on surgeon preference (**Figure 3-7**).

Postoperative Care

Routine wound care with gentle cleansing followed by application of a layer of antibiotic ointment are recommended. Cold compresses with ice or a Swedish mask are started in the recovery room and continued by the patient at home for at least 24 hours. A bag of frozen peas serves nicely in this function when the patient is at home. Patients are instructed to limit their physical activities to avoid heavy lifting, bending, or straining for 2 weeks postoperatively. Patients return on postoperative days 5–7 for suture removal. Patients may resume contact lens use 2 weeks after surgery.

Complications

Fortunately, major complications such as hematoma or blindness are rare following upper blepharoplasty. Although typically associated with lower

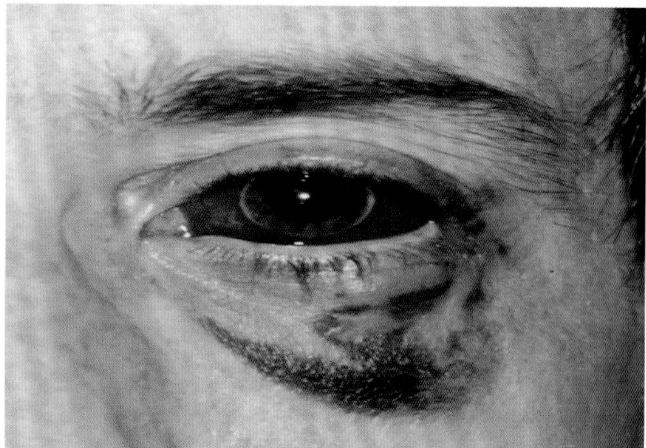

Figure 3-8. Orbital hematoma.

blepharoplasty, orbital hemorrhage with visual loss is possible in upper blepharoplasty. This must be considered in patients complaining of severe acute orbital pain who present with proptosis, chemosis, and ophthalmoplegia. Management of this possible catastrophic problem includes emergency exploration of the surgical site with possible hematoma evacuation. A lateral canthotomy with cantholysis may be necessary if globe pressure remains elevated despite wound exploration (**Figure 3-8**).

Minor complications such as ecchymosis, eyelid edema, and lagophthalmos usually resolve spontaneously early in the postoperative period. Minor revision procedures may be required in the case of persistent fat, excess skin, or the appearance of milia along the scar. Persistent lagophthalmos may require skin grafting if not improved by time and massage (**Figures 3-9 and 3-10**).

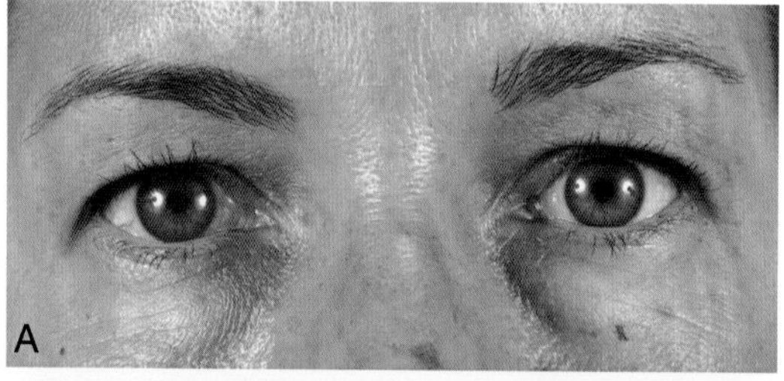

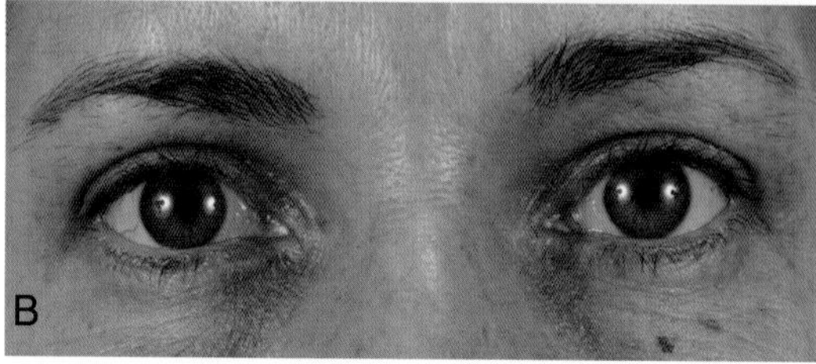

Figure 3-9. (A) Preoperative photo. (B) One-year postoperative photo.

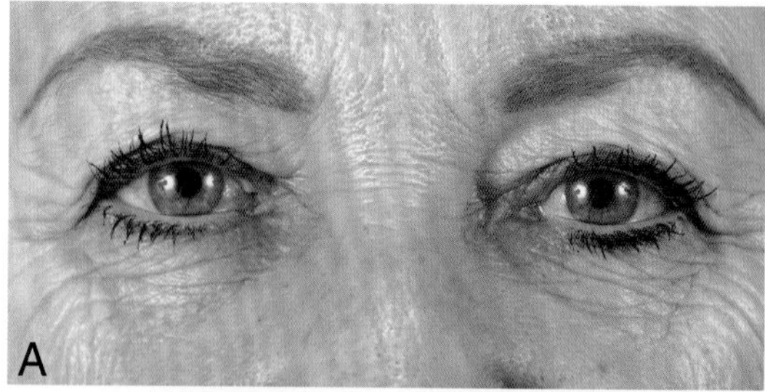

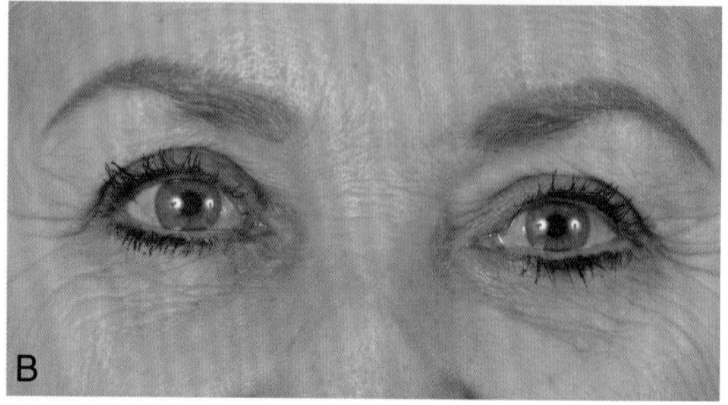

Figure 3-10. (A) Preoperative photo. (B) One-year postoperative photo.

Suggested Readings

1. Gentile RD. Upper lid blepharoplasty. *Facial Plast Surge CLIM N Am* 2005;13:511–524
2. Most SP, Mobley SR, Farabee WF. Anatomy of the eyelids. *Facial Plast Surge Clin N Am* 2005;13:487
3. Halvorson EG, Husni NR, Pandya SN, et al. Optimal parameters for marking upper blepharoplasty incisions. *Ann Plast Surg* 2006;56:569
4. Har-Shai Y, Hirshowitz B. Extended upper blepharoplasty for lateral hooding of the upper eyelid using a scalpel-shaped excision: A 13-year experience. *Plast Reconstr Surg* 2003;113:1028
5. Rohrich RJ, Coberly MC, Fagien S, et al. Current concepts in aesthetic upper blepharoplasty. *Plast Reconstr Surg* 2004;113:32e.
6. Fagien S. Advanced rejuvenative upper blepharoplasty: Enhancing aesthetics of the upper periorbita. *Plast Reconstr Surg* 2002;110:278
7. Pastorek NJ. Upper lid blepharoplasty. In Papel IP, ed. *Facial Plastic and Reconstructive Surgery,* 2nd ed. New York: Thieme Medical Publishers, 2002, p. 185
8. Daadat D, Dresner SC. Safety of blepharoplasty in patients with preoperative dry eyes. *Arch Facial Plast Surg* 2004;6:101
9. Persichetti P, Di Lella F, Delfino S, et al. Adipose compartments of the upper eyelid: Anatomy applied to blepharoplasty. *Plast Reconstr Surg* 2004; 113:373
10. Reid RR, Said HK, Yu M, et al. Revisiting upper eyelid anatomy: introduction of the septal extension. *Plast Reconstr Surg* 2006;117:65

4

Lower Eyelid Blepharoplasty

Theda C. Kontis, MD

Introduction

Aging of the lower eyelid is due to both descent of the malar complex as well as pseudoherniation of orbital fat. Patients complain that they look tired or their eyes look "puffy." In recent years, the procedure has undergone significant modifications. The first great advancement in lower blepharoplasty surgery was development of the transconjunctival approach, which reduced the incidence of postoperative ectropion and scarring. In addition, newer surgical techniques involve fat pad preservation and repositioning because traditional fat pad removal was noted to occasionally result in a hollow or sunken look. The fat preservation technique is used to camouflage the infraorbital rim, fill in the tear trough (nasojugal) depression, and provide a fuller, youthful lower-lid appearance.

Much like rhinoplasty, the key to successful lower blepharoplasty surgery is preoperative assessment. The facial plastic surgeon must be well versed in all the lower-lid operative techniques and select the correct procedures based on the anatomic findings of the individual patient.

Facial Analysis

Lower-Lid Anatomy

Evaluate the position and symmetry of the lower-lid margins. Note the presence of ectropion, increased roundin,g or scleral show. These indicate weakness of the lower lid, and consideration must be given for a lid-tightening procedure. Unrecognized lower-lid laxity is the most common cause of postoperative ectropion.

Evaluate the location and amount of pseudoherniated fat. This is the most common defect addressed with lower-lid blepharoplasty. The globe can be balloted, and the fat will herniate anteriorly. The fat is also demonstrated by having the patient gaze upward. On lateral view, the patient is assessed for a "double convexity" contour deformity, prominence of the herniated fat, and the malar mound (**Figure 4-1**).

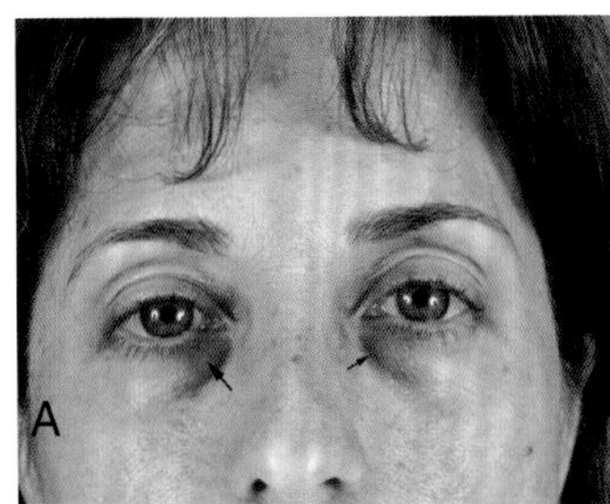

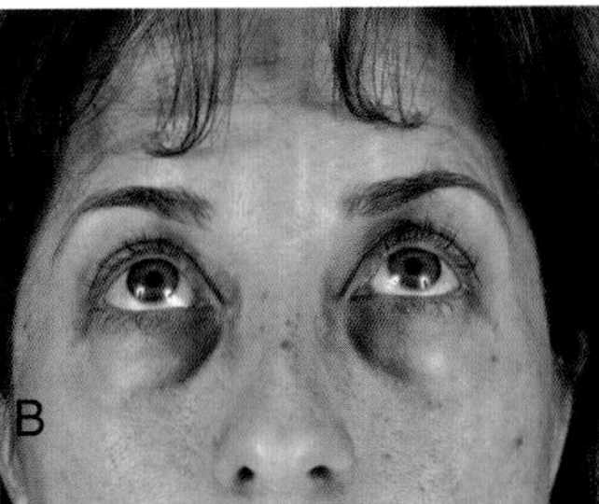

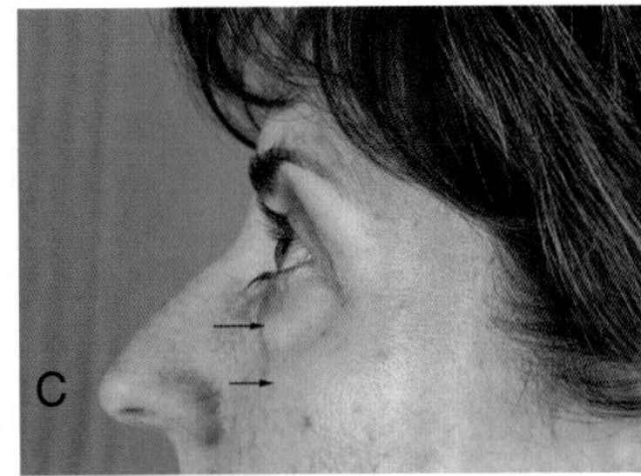

Figure 4-1. (A) Preoperative examination. Large arrow demonstrates pseudoherniation of lower lid fat. Small arrow marks the nasojugal groove or "tear trough" deformity. (B) Fat herniation is accentuated by upward gaze. (C) The "double convexity" contour deformity seen on lateral view results from prominences of herniated orbital fat and the descended malar mound (arrows).

Evaluate the presence and extent of the tear trough deformity or nasojugal groove (**Figure 4-1**). The nasojugal groove is a furrow which extends from the medial canthus inferiorly along the orbital rim. A deep tear trough deformity can be improved with either filler injections, or lower blepharoplasty with fat preservation and transposition. Fat repositioning may be performed through either a subciliary or transconjunctival approach.

Determine the amount of excess lower eyelid skin/bags. If minimal to no lower-lid skin needs to be excised, then a transconjunctival approach can be selected. If necessary, a skin pinch excision, chemical peel, or laser skin resurfacing may be performed concomitantly. If significant skin must be excised, then a subciliary incision is chosen.

The contribution of hypertrophic orbicularis oculi muscle to the lower-lid "bag" must be clarified preoperatively. Failure to recognize the hypertrophic muscle can be a pitfall of lower-lid blepharoplasty. The surgeon must recognize the difference between pseudoherniated fat and hypertrophic orbicularis muscle (**Figure 4-2**). Having the patient squint will bunch up the muscle if the "bag" is due to the hypertrophic orbicularis muscle. If this is so, it is the orbicularis muscle, not fat, that will need to be excised. Alternatively, botulinum toxin can be injected into the hypertrophic orbicularis muscle; however, this may result in increased scleral show.

Preoperative Considerations

General Health

As in any surgery, the general health of the patient must be assessed. The medical history should be reviewed, and the risk for anesthesia evaluated.

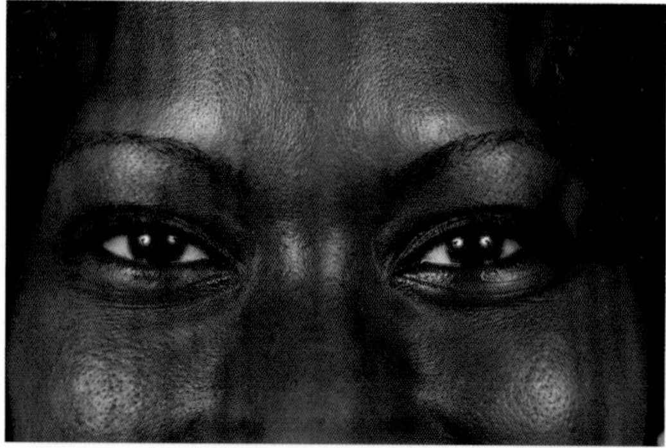

Figure 4-2. Hypertrophic orbicularis muscle accentuated by smiling or squinting. Note how this compares to the herniated fat seen in Figure 4-1A.

The patient's medication list should be discussed. The patient should not be taking anticoagulants or nonsteroidal anti-inflammatory medications for 2 weeks prior to surgery, including aspirin, ibuprofen, warfarin (Coumadin), and clopidrogel bisulfate (Plavix).

Ocular Health

The patient's general eye health should be discussed. Does the patient have any ophthalmological diseases or visual problems? Does the patient have dry eyes? A Schirmer's test can be performed to evaluate for dry eye. If the tear film travels less then 10 mm in 5 minutes, the patient has significant xerophthalmia. Although this is not an absolute contraindication to surgery, it should be recognized preoperatively. If there are any concerns about the patient's ophthalmologic health, an ophthalmology consult should be obtained preoperatively.

Lower-Eyelid Strength

The strength of the lower lid must be evaluated. The snap test or distraction test is performed by pulling the eyelid downwards and evaluating how long it takes the lid to "snap" back into its original position. If the skin returns slowly, or if the patient must blink to allow the lid to return to its original position, then lower-lid laxity is present. The pinch test is performed by pinching the lower lid away from the globe and seeing how quickly the lid again reapproximates the globe. Delays in return to baseline alert the surgeon that a lid-tightening procedure should be considered.

Preoperative Photographs

Photographic documentation should be performed both pre- and post-operatively. Classic views include full face, close up of eyes, eyes with upward gaze, lateral and oblique views (**Figure 4-3**). During the surgical procedure, it is useful to have the preoperative photographs displayed in the operating room.

Planning Surgery

Once the patient has been examined, the surgeon should outline the operative plan. The surgical approach is determined by the amount of excess lower-lid skin. The decision to remove or preserve fat is dictated by the presence of a tear trough deformity. Finally, a tarsal suspension must be considered to tighten a weak lower lid (**Figure 4-4**).

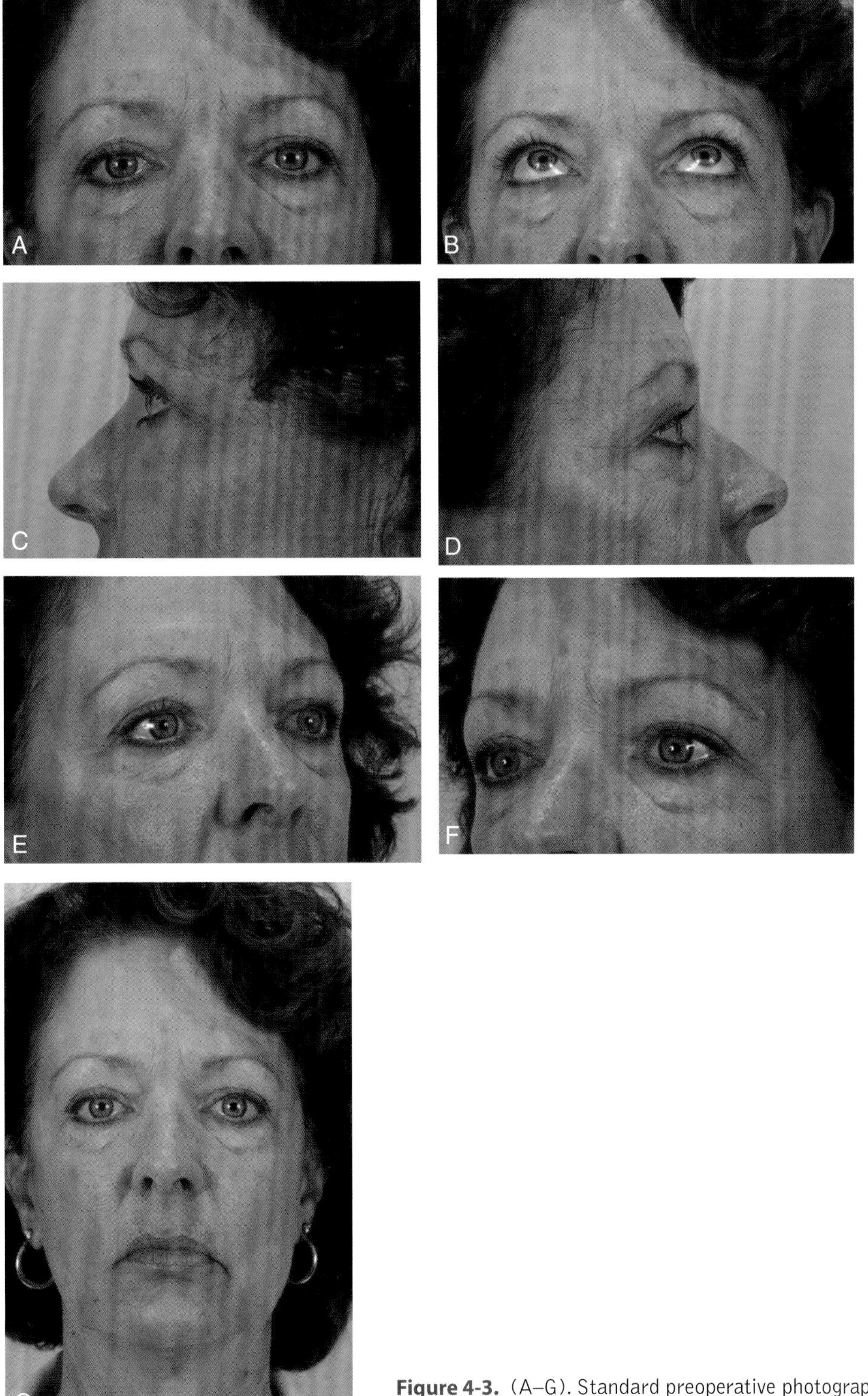

Figure 4-3. (A–G). Standard preoperative photographic views for blepharoplasty.

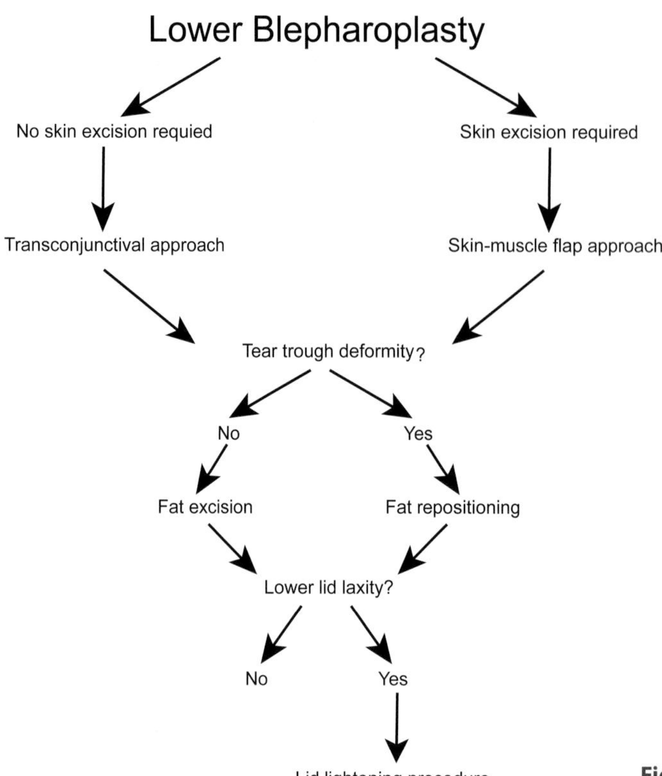

Figure 4-4. Lower Blepharoplasty Algorithm.

Consent

A preoperative discussion with the patient should include description of the risks of surgery. These may include: injury to the eye, diplopia, change in lower-lid position, asymmetry, scarring and the need for revision surgery. As in any cosmetic procedure, it is crucial that the patient have realistic expectations for the surgical results.

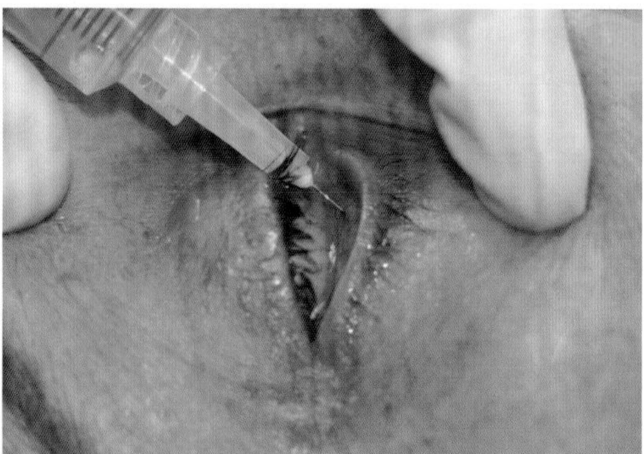

Figure 4-5. Injection of local anesthetic.

Technique

Transconjunctival Approach with Fat Excision

General anesthesia or intravenous sedation may be used.

Local anesthesia (Lidocaine 1% with 1:100,000 epinephrine) is infiltrated using a 30-gauge needle (**Figure 4-5**). If the patient is sedated, a drop of tetracaine ophthalmic solution is placed in each eye prior to injection.

Surgeon stands or seated at head of patient, essentially working "upside down."

A retractor is placed on lower lid with care being taken not to injure the lid margin (**Figure 4-6**).

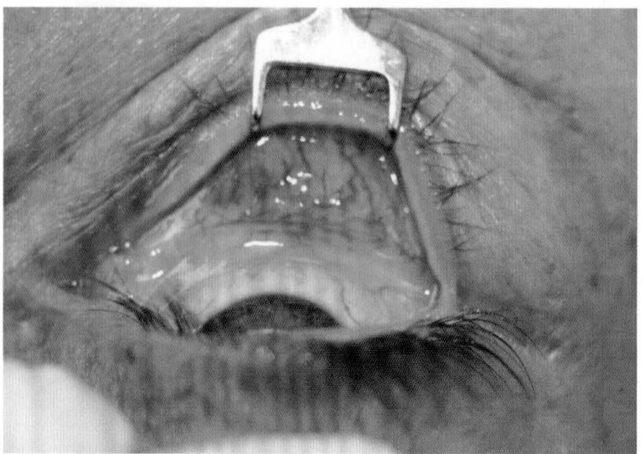

Figure 4-6. The lower eyelid vascular arcade.

Cautery used to make incision just below vascular arcade at the inferior edge of the tarsus

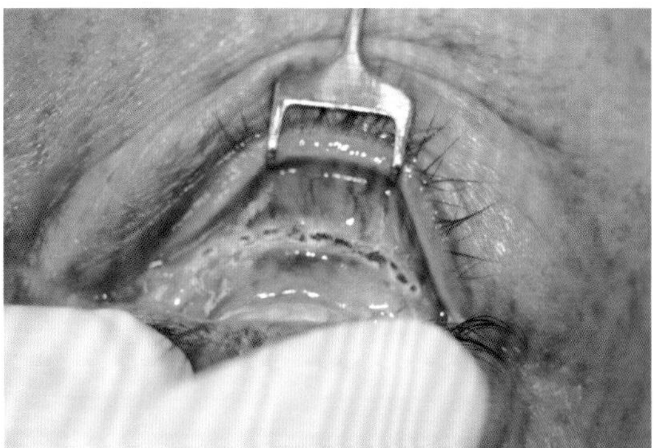

Figure 4-7. Cautery incision in created at the inferior aspect of the vascular arcade.

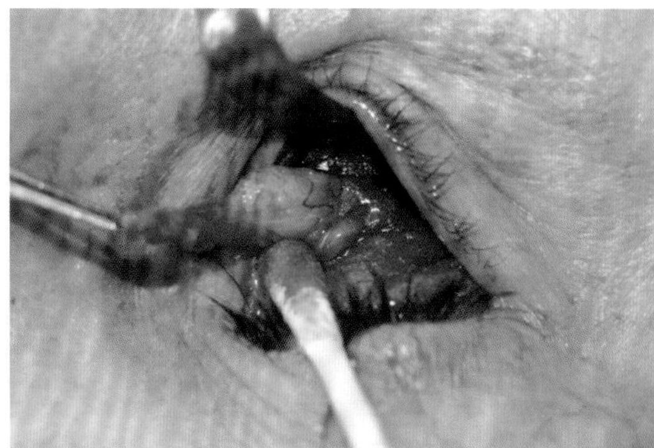

Figure 4-9. The fat pads are gently teased away from the surrounding tissue.

(**Figure 4-7**). The incision is then opened by using the electrocautery or by spreading with scissors.

The lower flap is retracted by using a 5-0 Nylon, held loosely with a clamp, which serves to provide counter-traction to facilitate dissection (**Figure 4-8**).

As the dissection proceeds inferiorly, pushing on the globe will allow the fat pads to bulge forward, which aids in identification of lower-lid fat compartments. The central fat pocket is usually encountered first. The fascia surrounding fat is divided to allow the fat to be expressed. The fat is gently teased away from the fibrous tissue using a cotton tipped applicator (**Figure 4-9**). Care must be taken not to exert excessive pull on the fat pad causing avulsion, which could result in an orbital hemorrhage.

The fat pad is cauterized with bipolar electrocautery and excised (**Figure 4-10**). To prevent a retrobulbar hematoma, it is imperative that bleeding be well controlled before the fat is released and allowed to retract back into the orbit. In addition, fat must not be overresected. A general rule is to gently remove what expresses easily and not remove fat deeper than the level of the inferior orbital rim.

The lateral pad is dissected and cauterized and removed. Gentle pressure on the globe allows excess fat to be identified.

The medial pad is identified next. The inferior oblique muscle can be seen to lie between the medial and central fat pads (**Figure 4-11**). The fat in the medial compartment is white or pale yellow when compared to the bright yellow fat of the central and lateral compartments. If the patient is under sedation, he or she may experience pain in this area, and the medial pad may require injection of additional local anesthetic. Traction on the medial fat pad can result in bradycardia due to the oculocardiac reflex. When dissecting the medial fat pad, it is helpful to notify the anesthesiologist of a possible bradycardic response. Release of traction will improve the reflex bradycardia.

The 5-0 nylon retraction suture is released and the tissue allowed to redrape. The lower lid is

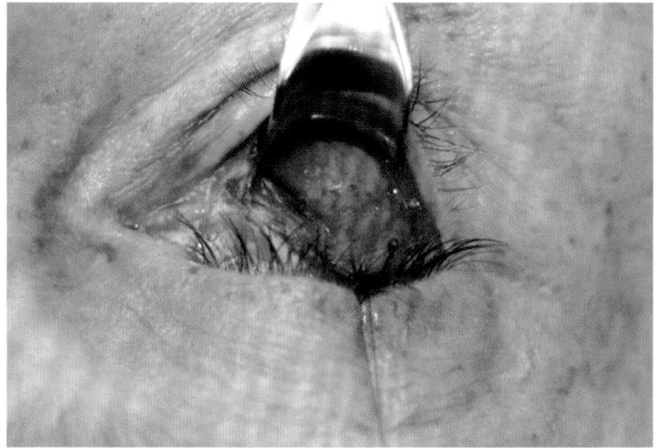

Figure 4-8. A suture is placed in the inferior flap and clamped with a needle holder to allow counter-traction during the dissection.

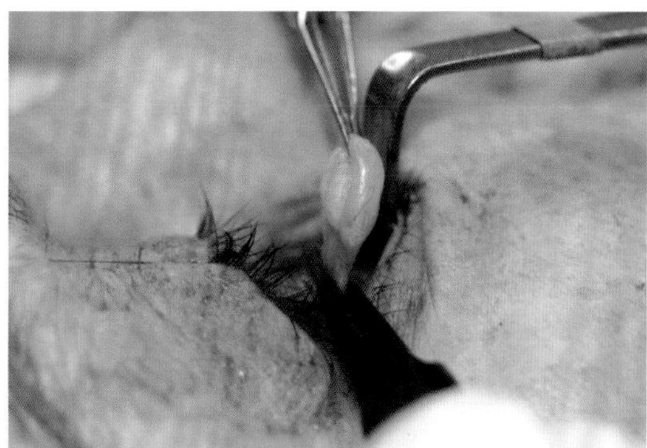

Figure 4-10. The lateral, central and medial fat pads are cauterized and excised.

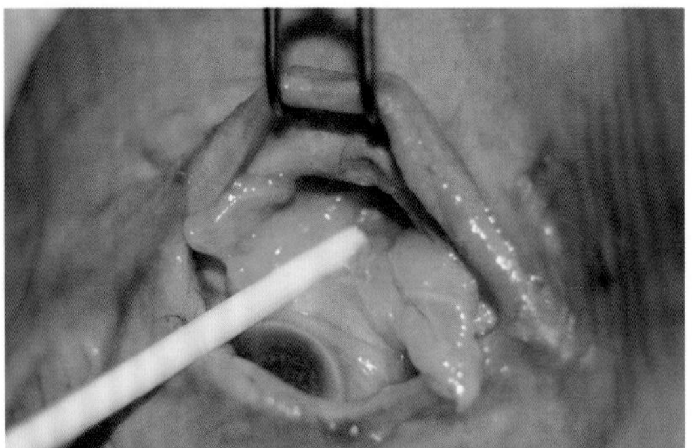

Figure 4-11. The instrument points towards the location of the inferior oblique muscle in a cadaveric specimen. The muscle is located between the medial and central fat pad compartments.

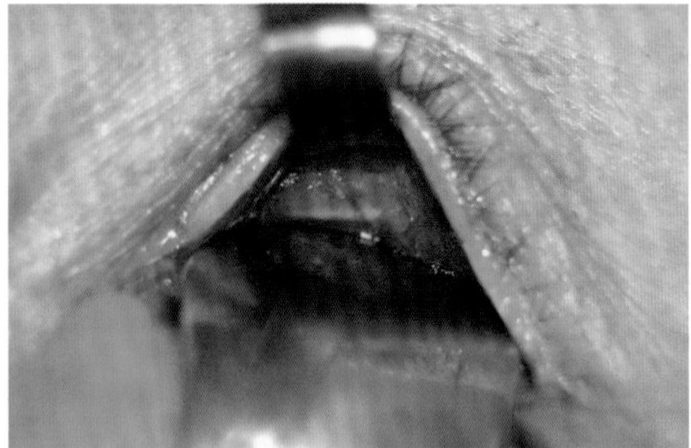

Figure 4-12. A Jaeger lid plate retractor is used to retract the dissected fat pads, and to allow visualization of the arcus marginalis: seen here as the white band of tissue at the tip of the retractor plate.

assessed for any retained fat. No sutures are placed in the transconjunctival incision.

Occasionally a skin pinch excision is performed when a small amount of excess skin is present. A small hemostat is used to squeeze the skin together just underneath the lash line. This standing ridge of pinched skin is excised using Westcott scissors. The incision is closed with interrupted 6-0 fast absorbing gut suture. Only about 2–3 mm of skin is excised using this technique. Resurfacing of the lower-lid skin also may be performed concomitantly, as no undermining of the skin was performed.

Transconjunctival Approach with Fat Preservation

Preoperative markings may be placed along the tear–trough depression to aid in correct intraoperative placement of the fat pedicle.

The transconjunctival approach is performed as outlined above and the lateral fat pad is removed.

The medial and central pads are dissected free. If the pedicle is too wide to allow easy rotation inferiorly, the pedicle may be narrowed using the electrocautery, with care being taken not to injure the blood supply.

The inferior orbital rim is exposed and the gleaming white arcus marginalis identified (**Figure 4-12**). The arcus marginalis is defined as the confluence of the orbital septum and periosteum of the maxilla. The electrocautery is used to divide the periosteum at the level of the arcus marginalis and a Freer Elevator is used to create a subperiosteal pocket (**Figure 4-13**). Careful dissection prevents injury to the infraorbital nerve.

Depending on the amount of fat available and the depth of the deformity, either the medial or

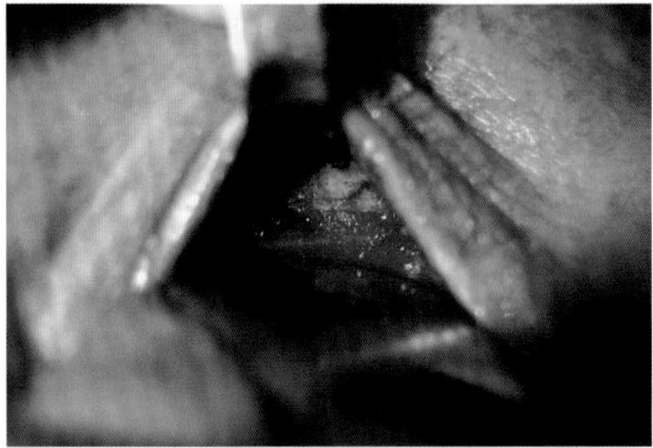

Figure 4-13. The electrocautery is used to score the periosteum at the arcus marginalis and an elevator used to create a subperiosteal pocket.

medial and central fat pedicles are draped over the infraorbital rim and tucked into the subperiosteal pocket. The fat should occupy the site indicated by the preoperative marking of the tear–trough deformity.

A 5-0 polyglactin (Vicryl) suture is used to secure fat in the subperiosteal pocket (**Figure 4-14**). A small bit of periosteum is taken from inside the subperiosteal pocket. The fat is positioned in the pocket and the suture is gently tied (**Figure 4-15**). Alternatively, a percutaneous nylon suture may be placed and removed several days postoperatively.

After suture fixation of the fat, a forced duction test is performed to ensure no entrapment of the inferior rectus muscle (**Figure 4-16**).

Subciliary Approach with or without Fat Repositioning

The procedure is performed under general or intravenous sedation anesthesia.

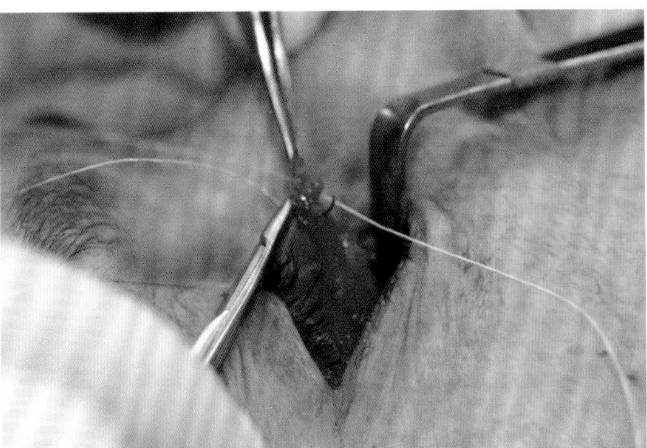

Figure 4-14. An absorbable suture is placed through and through the fat pedicle, and a small bite of periosteum is taken within the subperiosteal pocket.

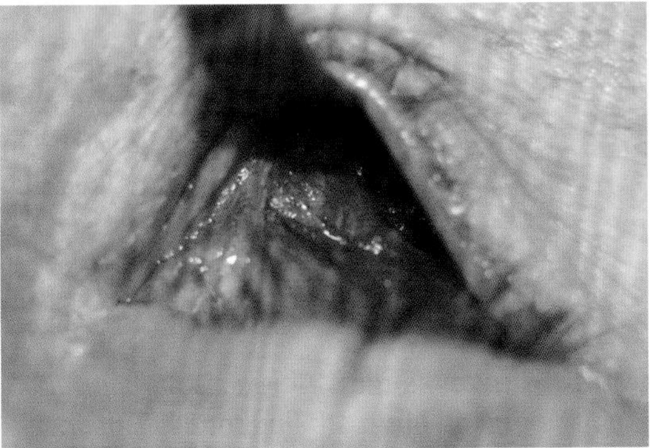

Figure 4-15. The suture is gently tightened, and the fat pedicle is secured into the subperiosteal pocket, in effect, camouflaging the infraorbital rim.

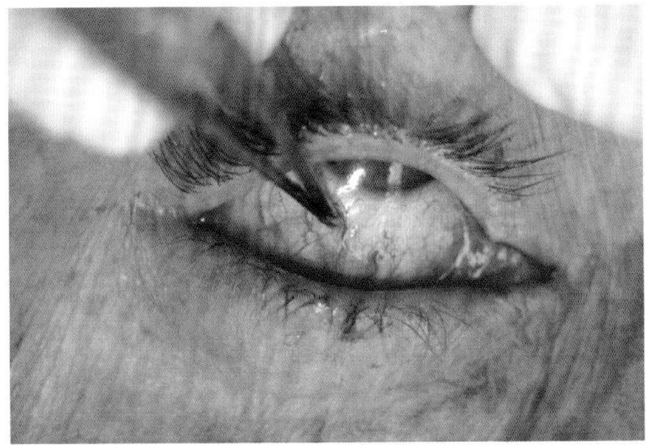

Figure 4-16. A forced duction test is performed to ensure no muscle entrapment has occurred after suture fixation.

Local anesthesia (1% Lidocaine with 1:100,000 epinephrine) is infiltrated using a 30-gauge needle.

The surgeon is positioned at the head of the patient so the procedure is performed "upside down."

A stab incision is made in the lateral canthal region (**Figure 4-17**) and Westcott scissors is used to undermine and incise the skin just below the gray line. The incision is extended just lateral to the tear duct punctum.

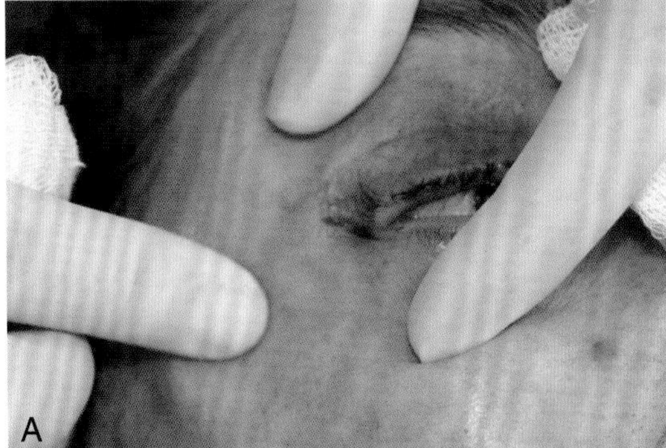

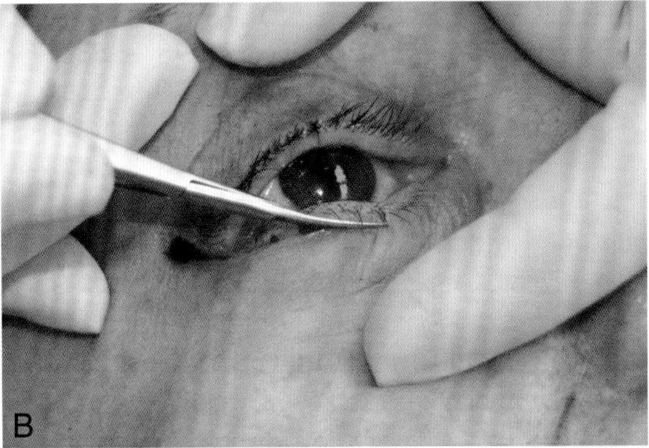

Figure 4-17. (A) Stab incision made at the lateral canthus. (B) Wescott scissors are used to complete the subciliary incision.

A traction suture of 5-0 nylon may be used to retract the lid superiorly. Dissection is carried out in the subcutaneous plane for a few millimeters, then the submuscular plane is entered. The remainder of the elevation is just deep to the orbicularis muscle, creating a "skin–muscle" flap.

Submuscular dissection proceeds to the level of the bony infraorbital rim. (**Figure 4-18**).

The orbital fat compartments are easily identified and fat is gently teased away from the surrounding fibrous tissue, cauterized with the bipolar cautery, and excised. Care is taken to maintain meticulous hemostasis.

If orbital fat is to be preserved, the arcus marginalis is identified and the cautery is to divide the periosteum. A Freer Elevator is used to create a subperiosteal pocket. Fat is removed from the lateral compartment, and the medial and/or central compartment fat is dissected to form an elongated pedicle, rotated over the infraorbital rim, and tucked into the subperiosteal pocket. The fat is sutured to the periosteum with 5-0 polyglactin (Vicryl).

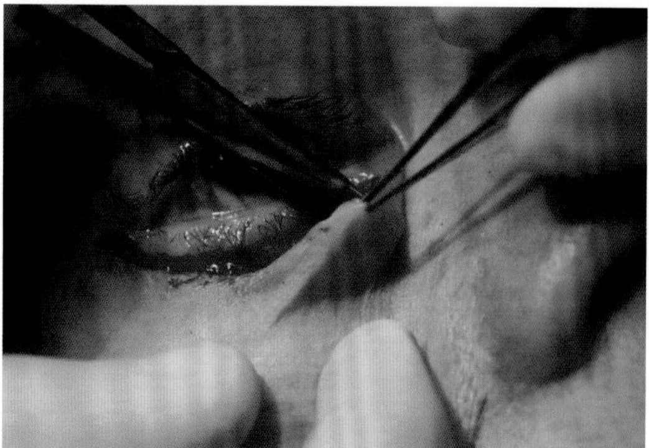

Figure 4-18. Dissection proceeds in the submuscular plane to the inferior orbital rim.

The skin is redraped on the lower eyelid and the traction suture released. If the patient is under sedation, he or she may be asked to open the mouth widely and look superiorly. This maneuver assists the surgeon in planning the amount of skin to excise. The skin flap is repositioned without tension and a conservative amount of skin is excised (**Figure 4-19**).

Once the skin is excised, orbicularis muscle is trimmed from the flap edge so that the closure reapproximates skin to skin. This maneuver prevents bunching of muscle at the incision line.

The skin is closed with a running or interrupted 6-0 fast absorbing gut suture (**Figure 4-20**).

Antibiotic ointment is applied to the suture line.

Tarsal Suspension

Many techniques exist for suspending the lateral canthus of a weak lower lid to prevent ectropion. The technique described here is a simple, versatile procedure used to support a lax lid but not to correct a gross ectropion deformity.

The premise of this technique is to suspend the lateral aspect of the tarsus to the medial aspect of the orbital rim.

Via the Transconjunctival Approach

After fat excision or transposition, a stab incision is made through the skin over the lateral aspect of the tarsus. If an upper blepharoplasty was performed concomitantly, the incision is left open until the canthopexy has been performed.

A 6-0 polypropylene (Prolene) or nylon suture is passed from the upper lid incision to the lower-lid incision, and passed through and through the lateral tarsus, the needle is then passed back to the upper lid incision. A bite of periosteum is taken along the

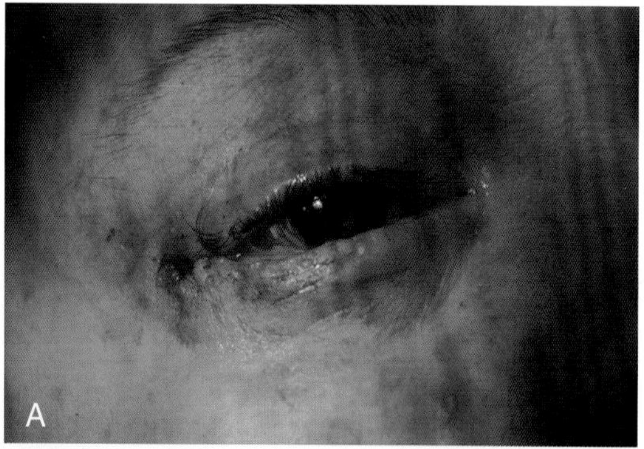

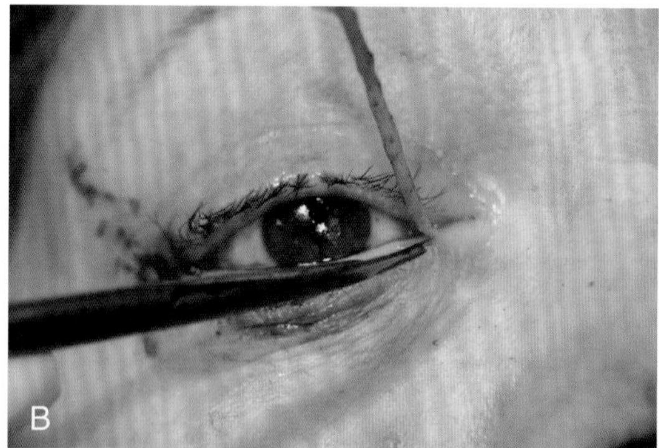

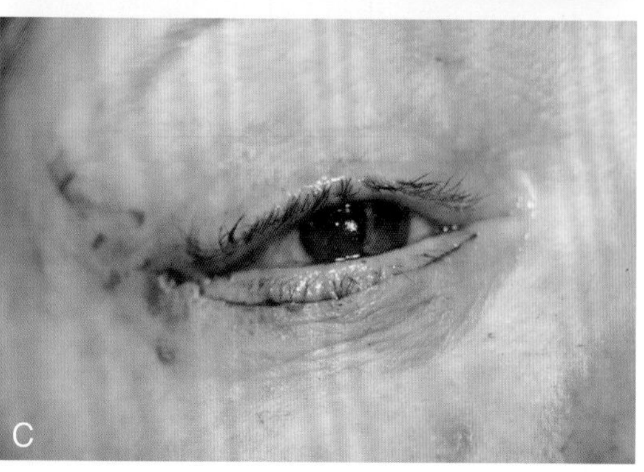

Figure 4-19. (A) The skin is redraped, and the patient is asked to open their mouth and/or to gaze upwards. (B) A conservative amount of skin is excised. (C) The lower lid after skin excision.

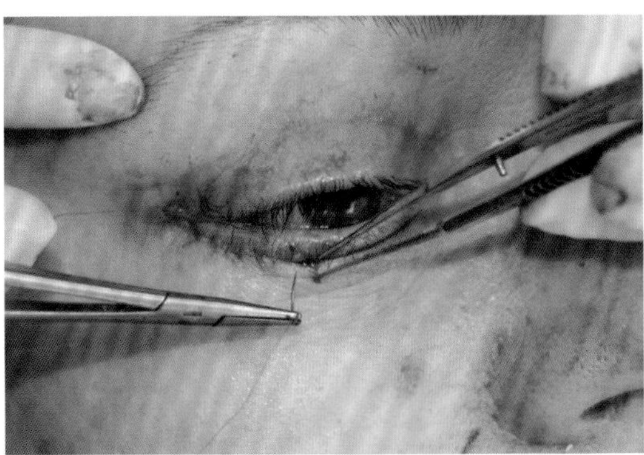

Figure 4-20. The incision is closed with a running or interrupted fast-absorbing suture.

medial aspect of the orbital rim. The suture is gently tightened, in order to slightly elevate the lateral canthus. The incisions are then closed in standard fashion.

Via skin-muscle flap approach

After fat excision or transposition, the lateral tarsus is visualized. A 6-0 polypropylene (Prolene) or Nylon suture is passed through and through the lateral tarsus. A firm bite of periosteum is taken along the medial aspect of the lateral orbital rim (**Figure 4-21**). The suture is tightened, which will raise the lateral canthus slightly. The incisions are closed.

Postoperative Care

In the immediate postoperative period, the patient's head is elevated, and iced compresses placed on the eyes.

Oral antibiotics and pain medication are prescribed.

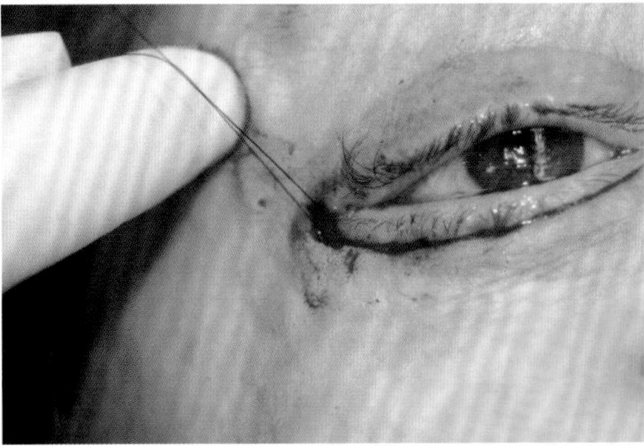

Figure 4-21. Lateral canthopexy is performed by placement of a permanent suture through the tarsal plate and lateral orbital rim (medial aspect) periosteum.

Iced compresses should continue for the first 24 hours postoperatively. The patient should sleep with their head elevated on two pillows for at least one week.

The eyes should be kept moist with preservative-free artificial tear drops. The patient is advised to not pull down lid margin when placing the drops.

Antibacterial ointment is prescribed for the subciliary suture line and should be applied three times a day.

The patient is advised to avoid strenuous activity for at least one week.

The patient is usually seen on the first postoperative day, to ensure no hematoma, loss of visual acuity or inferior rectus entrapment. If significant chemosis is present, steroid ophthalmic drops may be initiated.

The patient is seen again at one week postoperatively. No suture removal is required.

Post operative photography begins at the 6 week postoperative visit (**Figures 4-22, 4-23, 4-24, 4-25**).

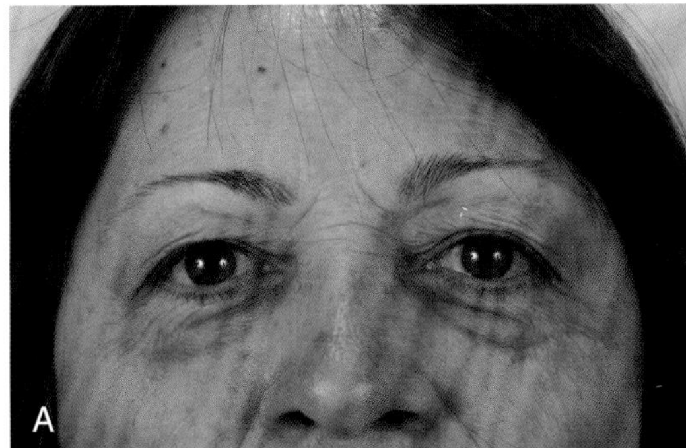

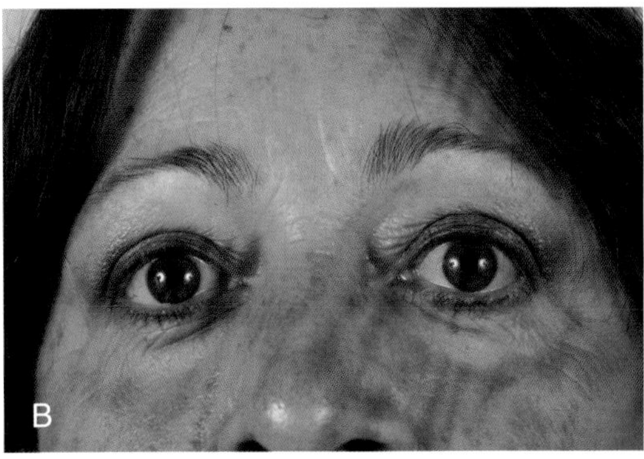

Figure 4-22. (A) Preoperative view demonstrating moderate orbital fat herniation, mild to moderate skin excess, and no significant nasojugal groove. (B) Post operative view. This patient underwent a transconjunctival lower blepharoplasty with fat removal and chemical peel of the lower lids. Upper blepharoplasty and endoscopic browlift were also performed.

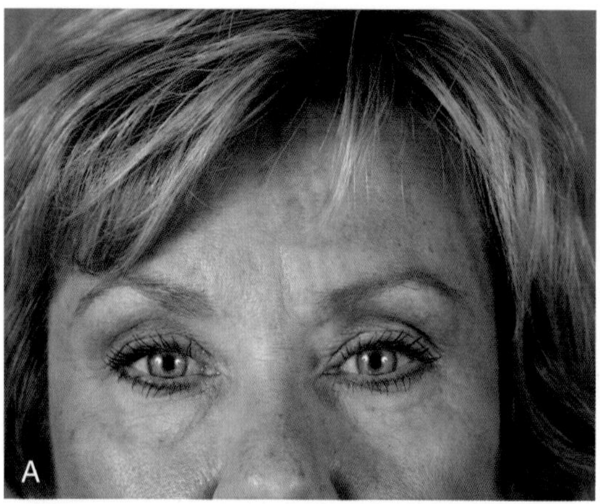

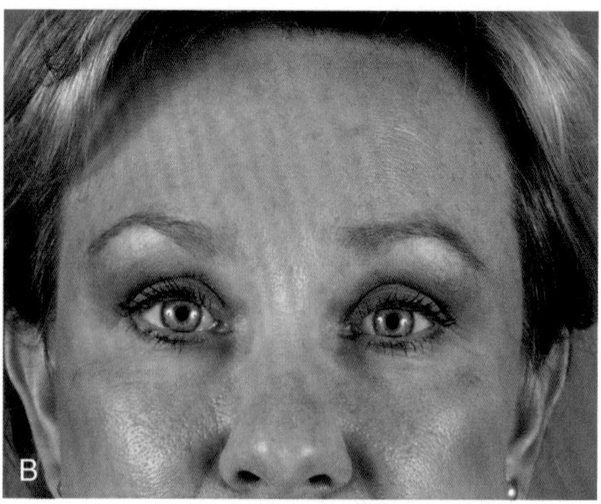

Figure 4-23. (A) Preoperative view demonstrating mild to moderate fat herniation, mild skin excess, and a moderately deep nasojugal groove. (B) Postoperative view after transconjunctival lower blepharoplasty with fat pad transposition and chemical peel of the lower lid skin. Upper blepharoplasty, endoscopic browlift and rhytidectomy were also performed.

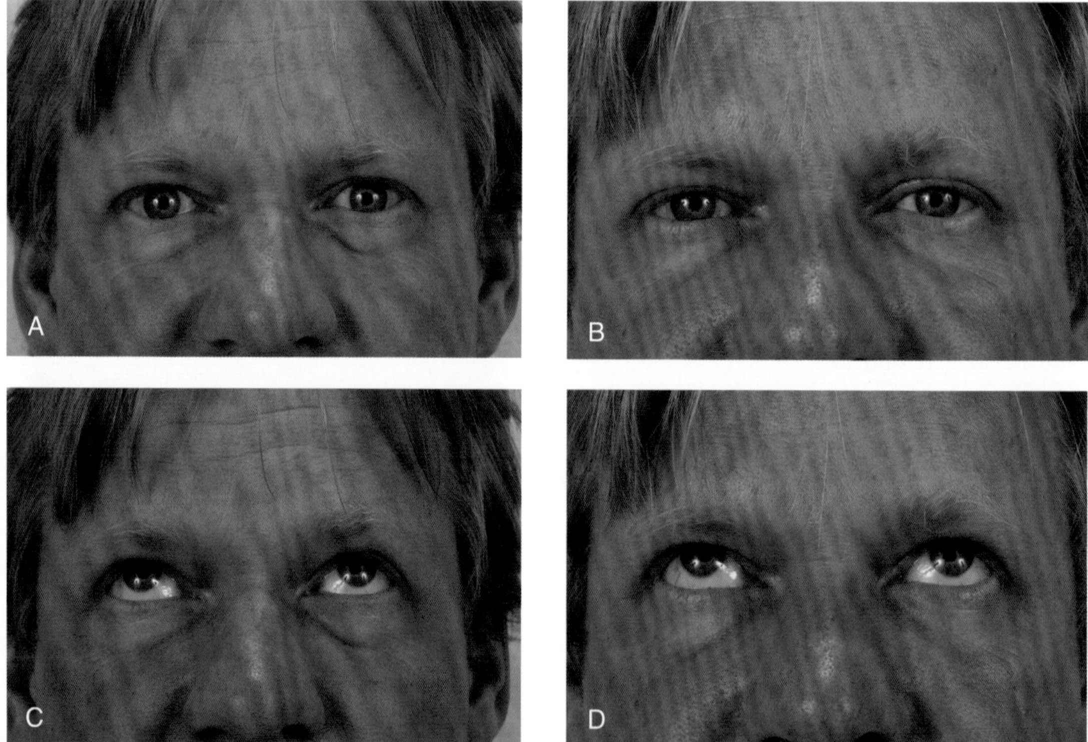

Figure 4-24. (A) Preoperative view demonstrating significant fat pad herniation, deep nasojugal grooves and moderate skin excess. (B) Fat pads are accentuated with upward gaze. (C, D) Postoperative views following transconjunctival lower blepharoplasty with fat pad repositioning.

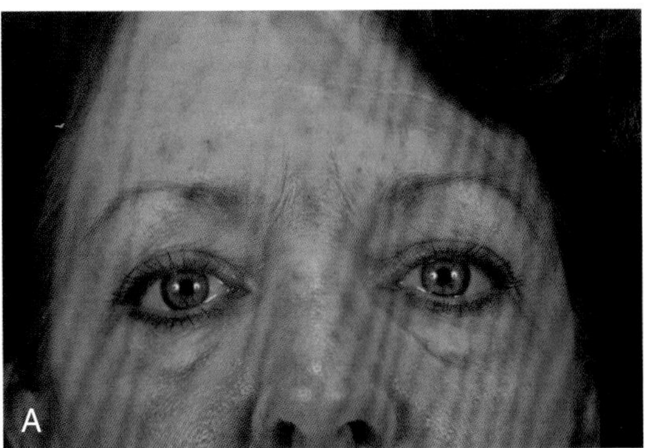

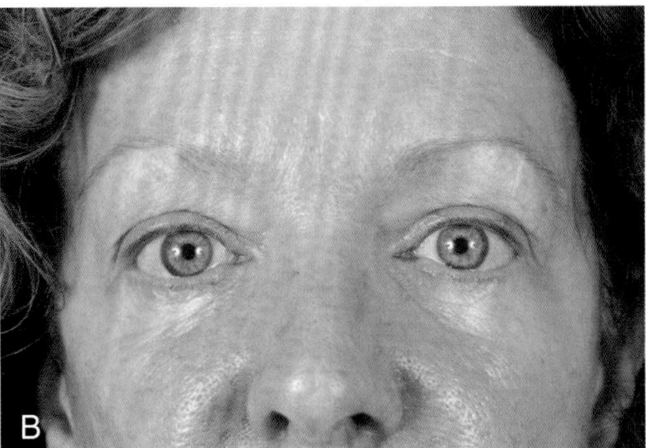

Figure 4-25. (A) Preoperative view of a patient with significant lower lid fat herniation, lax lower lids and excess lower lid skin without significant nasojugal grooves. (B) Postoperative view following subciliary lower blepharoplasty with fat excision and lateral tarsal suspension.

Complications

Hemorrhage: The most feared, and fortunately rare, complication of lower blepharoplasty is retrobulbar hematoma. Such hemorrhage may increase intraorbital pressure, which prevents retinal artery flow and blindness may follow. In lower-lid blepharoplasty, every attempt must be made to minimize bleeding: assessment and control of preoperative medications, meticulous intraoperative hemostasis, gentle emergence from anesthesia, and mandating that the patient have limited activity in the first postoperative week.

Ectropion: An undesirable but avoidable complication of blepharoplasty is ectropion (**Figure 4-26**). A diligent preoperative evaluation of lower-lid strength is important, and intraoperative tarsal suspension should be performed when lid laxity is noted. If ectropion appears to be developing in the postoperative period, upward massage of the lid and/or vertical taping may prevent or reduce its development.

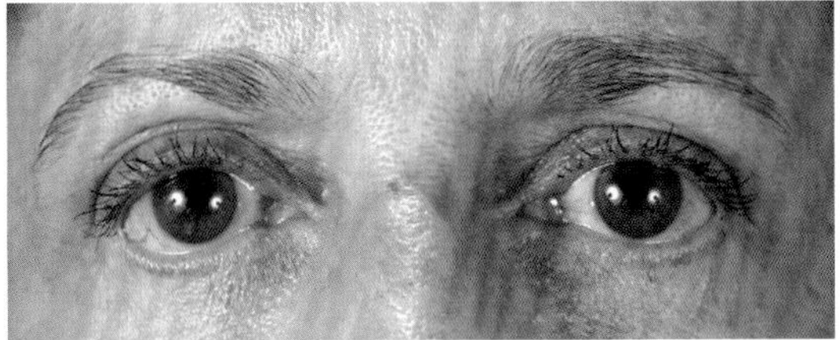

Figure 4-26. Postoperative ectropion likely due to subciliary approach with excessive skin excision and failure to perform a lid tightening procedure.`

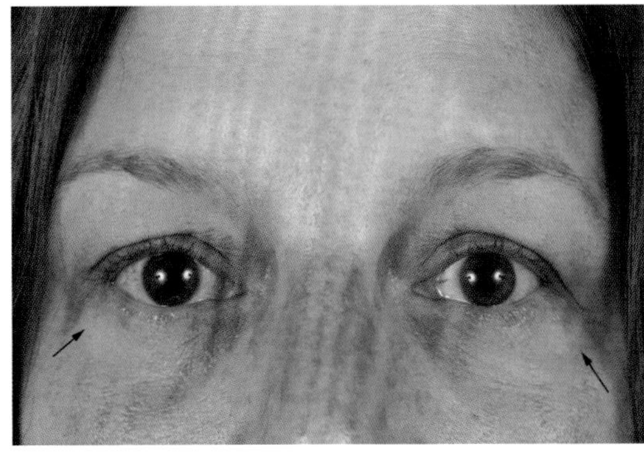

Figure 4-27. Arrows demonstrate retained lateral fat pads following transconjunctival blepharoplasty.

Retained fat pads: Common complications of lower-lid surgery include asymmetry and retained fat pads. Lower lids are not always symmetric, and subtle asymmetries should be pointed out to the patient preoperatively. Occasionally, inadequate fat removal will result in postoperative "lumps." The lateral compartment is the most common site of retained fat (**Figure 4-27**). This fat is easily addressed at a revision surgery, usually under local anesthesia through a transconjunctival approach.

Hyperpigmentation: Postoperative hyperpigmentation of the lower eyelid skin can occur in some patients (**Figure 4-28**). This is generally treated with hydroquinone and sunscreen.

Scarring: Scarring of subciliary incision is usually not an issue, unless the incision is placed too far inferiorly. In general, if the incision is kept close to the lash line, it heals with an imperceptible scar.

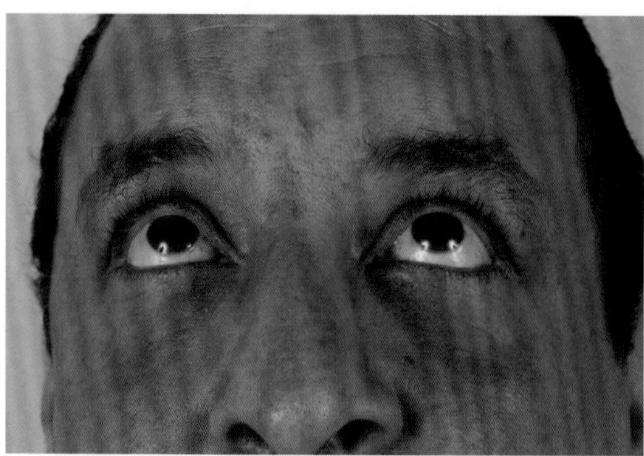

Figure 4-28. Hyperpigmentation seen after lower blepharoplasty.

Diplopia: A forced duction test is performed after fat repositioning, to alert the surgeon to possible entrapment of the inferior rectus muscle.

Lumpiness: Repositioned fat can sometimes be palpable along the tear-trough region in the early post-operative period. This is temporary and the patient should be aware this will resolve in time without treatment.

Suggested Readings

1. Garcia RE, McCollough EG. *Arch Facial Plast Surg* 2006;8(6):374–380.
2. Lee, AS and Thomas JR. "Lower Lid Blepharoplasty and canthal surgery." *Facial Plast Surg Clin N Am* 2005;13(4):541–551.
3. Marrone, AC. "Lower Eyelid blepharoplasty" In *Oculoplastic Surgery,* Ed Wright KW and Tse, DT. JB Lippincott, Philadelphia. 1992, p.189–200.
4. Mohadjer Y and Holds JB. "Cosmetic Lower Eyelid blepharoplasty With Fat Repositioning via Intra-SOOF Dissection: Surgical Technique and Initial Outcomes." *Ophthal Plast Reconstr Surg* 2006;22(6):409–413.
5. Nassif, PS. "Lower blepharoplasty: Transconjunctival Fat Repositioning." *Otolaryngol Clin N Am* 2007;40(2): 381–390.
6. Patipa, M. "The Evaluation and Management of Lower Eyelid Retraction following Cosmetic Surgery." *Plast Reconstr Surg* 2000;106(2):438–453.
7. Putterman AM. "Treatment of lower Eyelid Dermatochalasis, herniated Orbital Fat, Abnormal Appearing Skin, and hypertrophic Orbicularis Oculi Muscle: Skin Flap Approach" In Cosmetic Oculoplastic Surgery, WB Saunders, Philadelphia. 1999, p.179–193.

5

Management of Ectropion, Laxity, and Retraction in the Blepharoplasty Patient

Marc J. Hirschbein, MD, FACS and James Karesh, MD

It is important to identify ectropion and eyelid laxity during surgical evaluation of the blepharoplasty patient. Ectropion is a frequently encountered eyelid malposition. It is defined as the eversion or outward rotation of the eyelid margin away from the globe. Ectropion is far more common in the lower lid than the upper lid. It can be classified as congenital, mechanical, involutional, cicatricial, tarsal, or paralytic. Lower lid retraction is defined as a vertical shortening of the lower lid in relation to the globe. Lower lid retraction may be present preoperatively, and it is one of the more feared complications following lower eyelid blepharoplasty. Evaluation and management of this entity will be addressed in the second part of this chapter.

There are six anatomic factors that contribute to ectropion. They may occur alone or in combination. These include horizontal eyelid laxity, medial canthal tendon laxity, punctual malposition, vertical tightness or shortening of the skin, orbicularis oculi paresis, and inferior lid retractor disinsertion. Successful surgical repair depends on identifying and correcting the causative anatomic defect or defects.

Anatomy

The lower eyelid can be divided into three layers. The anterior lamella includes the skin and orbicularis muscle. The middle lamella consists of the orbital septum and orbital fat. The capsulopalpebral fascia and conjunctiva make up the posterior lamella. Pathology in any of these layers will disrupt the anatomic equilibrium of the lid, resulting in eyelid malposition (**Figure 5-1**).

Unlike the upper eyelid, which has a distinct retractor in the levator muscle, the lower-lid retractor complex is less well defined. It begins as the capsulopalpebral head, a fascial extension of the inferior rectus muscle. This fascia splits to surround and fuse with the inferior oblique muscle sheath. It reunites to form Lockwood's ligament—the "lower suspensory ligament" of the globe. Anterior to Lockwood's ligament, the retractor complex is termed the capsulopalpebral fascia. A portion of this fascia inserts on the inferior fornix. Approximately 5 m below the inferior tarsal border, the capsulopalpebral fascia, orbital septum, and inferior tarsal muscle meet to form a single fascial layer that extends upward toward the tarsus. Some fibers extend through orbicularis fibers and skin to form

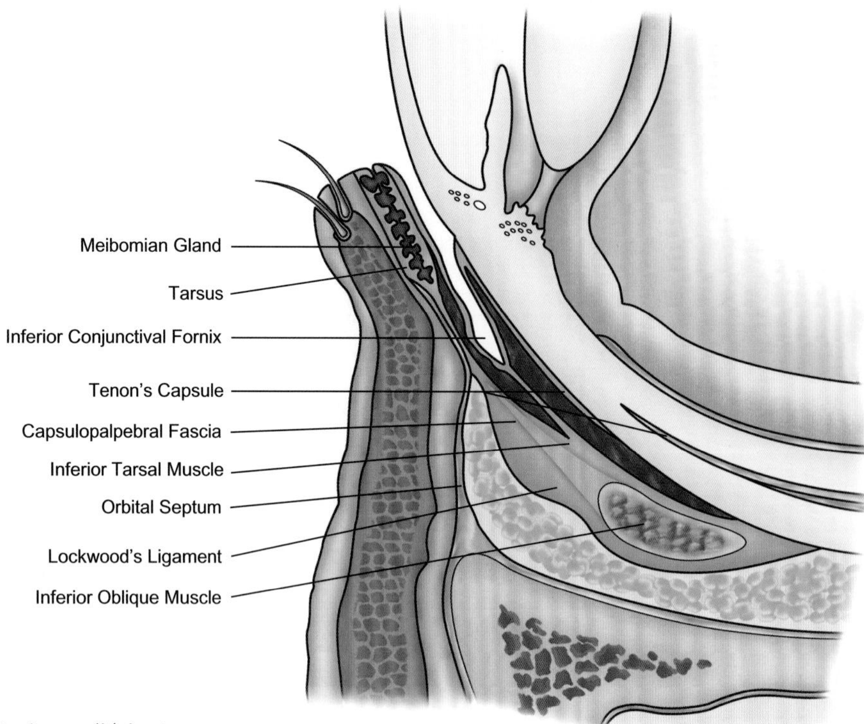

Figure 5-1. Lower-lid Anatomy.

the lower-lid crease. The smooth muscle fibers disappear 2 mm below the tarsus. The capsulopalpebral fascia terminates at the inferior tarsal border, attaching to the anterior and posterior surfaces. (**Figure 5-2**)

The tarsal ligamentous sling provides the primary support for the eyelids. Medially, the medial canthal tendon is composed of an anterior head that joins to the maxillary process of the frontal bone. The deep head inserts onto the posterior lacrimal crest. The lateral retinaculum results from the fusion of several components of the upper and lower lids, including the lateral canthal ligament, orbicularis fibers, and the lateral portions of both Whitnall's and Lockwood's ligaments. It has broad attachments to the orbital rim periosteum. The insertion on the inner aspect of the orbital rim allows the lids to approximate the globe. Consequently, the lateral retinaculum influences eyelid shape, tension, and position.

Classification

Congenital Ectropion

Congenital ectropion is a rare disorder that is usually caused by a vertical deficiency of lid skin. It is more often associated with other abnormalities such as blepharophimosis syndrome or Down syndrome.

Mechanical Ectropion

Mechanical ectropion results from a mechanical force that displaces the lower-lid margin away from the globe. Causes include a lid tumor weighing down the lid, a hematoma, extensive chemosis, or a large prosthesis that can push the lower lid outward (**Figure 5-3**).

Paralytic Ectropion

Paralytic ectropion is a sequela of a facial nerve palsy and orbicularis weakness. Common causes include Bell's palsy, Möbius syndrome, acoustic neuroma, parotid tumors, myasthenia gravis, Parkinson's disease, facial trauma, and iatrogenic damage. Loss of innervation to the orbicularis muscle results in decreased eyelid tone, and the lower-lid margin sags away from the globe. Other signs of a 7th-nerve palsy may include a lower brow on the affected side, an incomplete blink, poorly defined nasolabial folds and forehead furrows, and punctal eversion resulting in epiphora (**Figure 5-4**)

Cicatricial Ectropion

Systemic conditions that cause cicatricial skin changes and vertical shortening of the anterior lamella may lead to ectropion. Disorders include

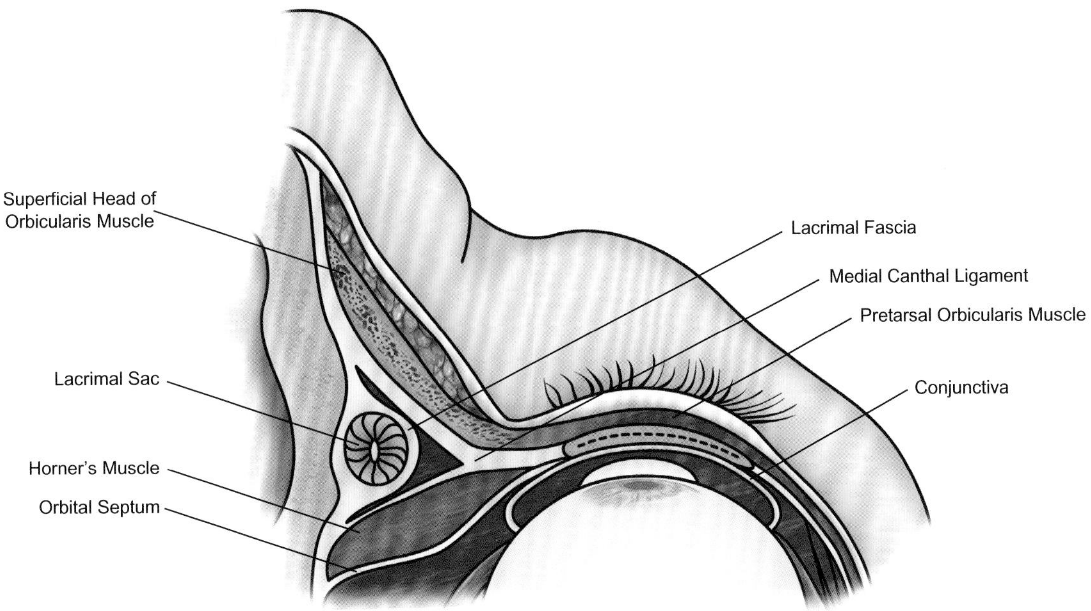

Figure 5-2. Horizontal view of lower-lid anatomy.

icthyosis, Stevens–Johnson syndrome, scleroderma, herpes zoster, and porphyria. Chronic atopic dermatitis, actinic damage, and burns (acid, alkali, and thermal) result in shortening of the anterior lamella. Frequently, ectropion develops postoperatively following blepharoplasty, rhytidectomy, chemical peels, or skin lesion excision.

Involutional Ectropion

Involutional ectropion is the most common type of ectropion. It is typified by horizontal eyelid laxity, involving the medial canthal tendon, lateral canthal tendon or both. Therefore, segmental or full lid eversion occurs. Patients may also have punctual ectropion causing epiphora and repeated wiping of tears. Skin excoriation and inflammation perpetuates the lid malposition.

Disinsertion of lower-lid retractors is another component of involutional ectropion. It may or may not be associated with horizontal laxity. The ensuing eyelid instability triggers tarsal ectropion, or complete eversion of the inferior tarsal plate. Signs include a deeper inferior fornix due to loss of capsulopalpebral fascial attatchments, a higher resting position of the lower lid, and decreased lid excursion from upgaze to downgaze.

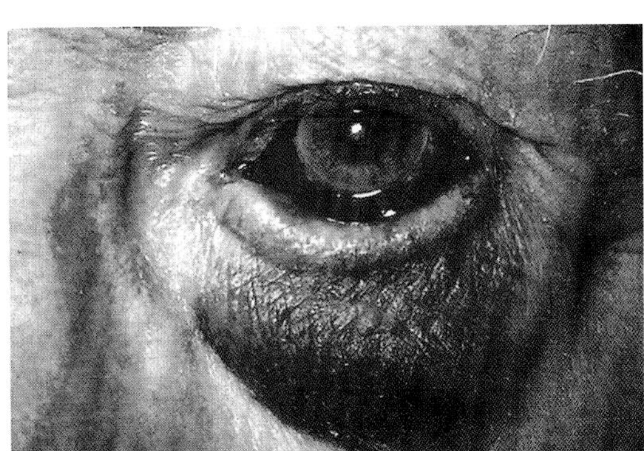

Figure 5-3. Mechanical ectropian secondary to hemorrhage.

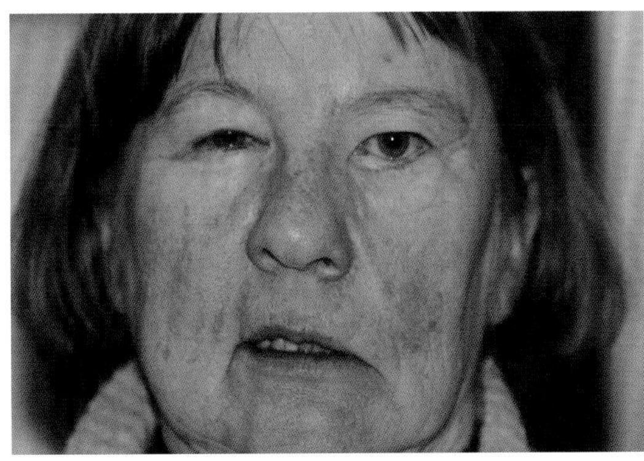

Figure 5-4. Paralytic ectropian secondary to mobius syndrome.

Evaluation

Assessment begins with observing the location and contour of the eyelids. Occasionally, a subtle ectropion can be seen on gross examination – as noted by a slight gap between the lower lid and the globe. The skin is examined for signs of inflammation and scarring. Laxity can best be evaluated by the "snap-back" test. The examiner pulls the lid downward away from the globe and then gently releases it. A normal lid will immediately snap back against the globe. A weakened lid will take several blinks to return to normal position and an ectropic lid will remain everted. Less often performed, the distraction test is then performed by gently pulling the central portion of the lower lid in an anterior-posterior direction. If 8 mm or more can be measured between the lid and globe, the lower lid is lax **(Figure 5-5)**. Medial canthal tendon laxity is present if the punctum can be drawn laterally past the nasal limbus. If laxity is present by any of these tests, the examiner should then attempt to bring the lateral canthus into position with one finger and assess the lower-lid position in relation to the inferior limbus. If the lid can be tightened horizontally, and the central lower lid is sitting at the desired vertical height (usually 1 mm above the inferior limbus), then the surgical plan should include some form of horizontal tightening (i.e., lateral tarsal strip or lateral suture canthopexy). If the central lower lid pulls below the inferior limbus while on horizontal stretch (requiring a second finger to elevate the lid centrally), then the surgical plan will also require a posterior or middle lamellar vertical graft (see below). This is a key preoperative distinction to make to ensure a successful surgical outcome. Finally, medial tendon laxity should be assessed. If the punctum can be pulled laterally to the pupil, the medial canthus will need to be tightened as well **(Figure 5-6)**. Failure to do so will often result in postoperative tearing due to canalicular stretch if only a lateral tightening procedure is employed.

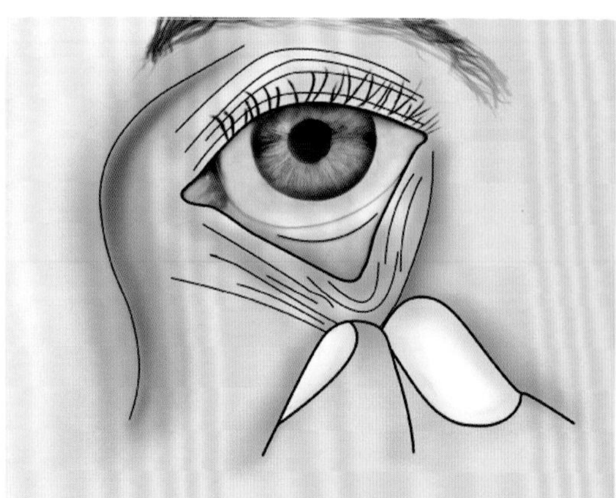

Figure 5-5. Distraction test and medial laxity.

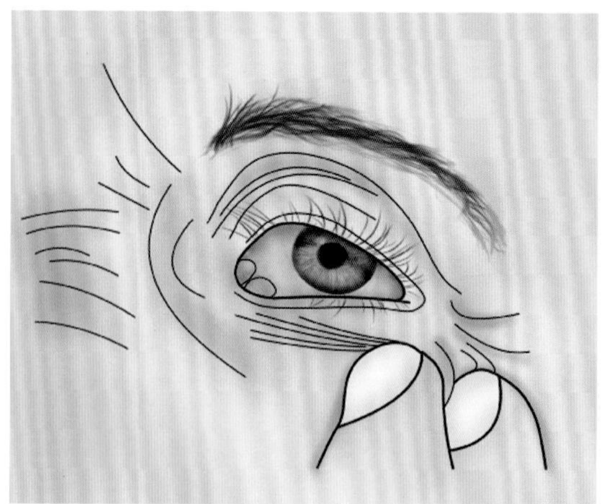

Figure 5-6. Distraction test and medial laxity.

Vertical excursion of the lower lid is then evaluated. Normally, the eyelid can easily be elevated to the pupil. In involutional ectropion with dehisced inferior retractors, the lower lid may extend beyond the superior limbus. On the other hand, in cicatricial ectropion, it is difficult to place the lid above the inferior limbus. If ectropion worsens with opening the mouth, or cheek and upper lip movement accompanies lid elevation, cicatricial changes are present.

Punctal position is also evaluated. The punctum should normally sit in apposition to the globe. If punctal ectropion is present and not addressed, tearing may result. If tearing is present preoperatively, the lacrimal system should be irrigated to rule out obstruction. Finally, if indicated, the conjunctiva is examined for inflammation and keratinization and the cornea is checked for keratopathy.

Surgical Management

Ectropion usually requires surgical management. The goals of surgery are to restore normal eyelid anatomy, recover lid function, and to protect the cornea from exposure keratopathy. Improved cosmesis is also expected. The next section will approach the surgical repair of lower eyelid laxity in the context of lower eyelid blepharoplasty. Surgical options will proceed from least to most severe.

Mild Lower-Eyelid Laxity

Evaluation: "Mild" laxity can be defined by the following criteria: (a) no frank ectropion visible on exam, (b)"snap-back" test with mild laxity (lid will slowly return to normal position no later than by the first blink) and/or distraction test less than 4 mm, (c) no vertical shortening or cicatricial components.

Surgical Repair: Lateral Canthopexy

This procedure should be performed towards the end of a lower eyelid blepharoplassty. If the blepharoplasty was transconjunctival, with no skin removal, a small (5 mm) incision should be made 1 mm subciliary at the lateral portion of the eyelid, and a small subcutaneous (or sub-orbicularis) pocket dissected inferiorly. If an upper blepharoplasty is also being performed, the canthopexy is performed prior to upper lid skin closure. If there is no planned upper blepharoplasty, a 5 mm incision should be made in the most lateral aspect of the upper eyelid lid crease.

A double-armed 4-0 or 3-0 suture (we prefer an absorbable Vicryl suture on a large curved cutting needle) is passed through the MOST LATERAL portion of the lower lid within the subcilliary pocket. The first needle is passed more superiorly, full thickness, through the lateral eyelid (engaging the lateral canthal tendon) – enters into the lateral orbit (avoiding the globe) – and is then directed superiorly and laterally engaging the periosteum on the *inner* edge of the *superior-lateral orbital rim* – and is then brought out through the upper lid incision. The second suture arm is placed 4 mm below the first arm, and follows a parallel path. Engaging tissue too medially will result in undesirable buckling of the lateral lid margin. Prior to tying, the sutures should be pulled upward and the lid position evaluated. If unacceptable (lateral canthus too high, buckled, or away from the globe) the suture should be cut and a new suture positioned. Care should be taken to avoid multiple passes or scraping along the periosteum – we have had one case referred in for retrobulbar hemorrhage from lateral canthopexy (**Figure 5-7**).

A

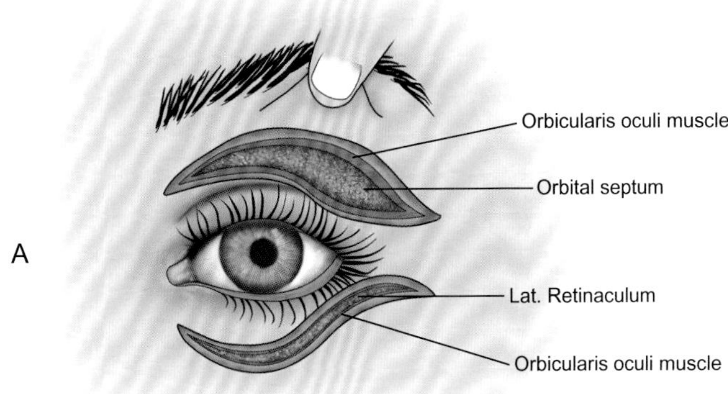

B

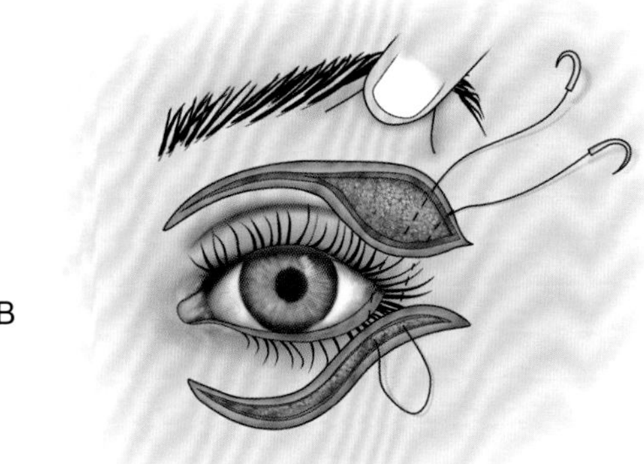

Figure 5-7. Lateral canthopexy.

Moderate Laxity to Frank Ectropion

Evaluation: "moderate" laxity can be defined by the following criteria: (a)no frank ectropion visible on exam, (b) "snap-back" test with moderate laxity (lid will not return to normal position until after the first one or two blinks) and/or distraction test greater than 4 mm and less than 8 mm, (c) no vertical shortening or cicatricial components. The following procedure is also appropriate for frank preoperative ectropion without cicatricial findings.

Surgical Repair: Lateral Tarsal Strip

Two to 3 cc of Lidocaine 2% with epinephrine 1:100,000, mixed 50:50 with Marcaine $^{1}/_{2}$% and optional sodium bicarbonate. Wydase is injected in the lateral canthal area subcutaneously to the inner aspect of the lateral orbital rim and into the deeper planes of the lateral lower eyelid. A lateral canthotomy is created with a #15 blade, Stevens scissors, or cutting cautery. The lateral lower lid is grasped with tooth forceps and pulled superiorly and laterally. The inferior crus of the lateral canthal tendon is strummed with scissors or cautery and the tight fibers are cut in an inferior nasal direction. Releasing the inferior crus creates a freely mobile lower lid. The edge of the lid is grasped with a forceps and drawn laterally. The wooden edge of a cotton-tipped applicator is placed on the lateral orbital rim. Where the applicator and the lid meet determines how much of the lid needs to be shortened. This spot may be marked on the lid if desired. A full-thickness incision is then made just beneath the tarsus from the lateral wound edge to the point below where the lid margin had been previously marked. The lid is then split into an anterior and posterior lamella with scissors or a blade to the point marked. Skin and orbicularis are removed. The mucocutaneous lid margin is also removed, taking care not to remove a portion of the tarsal plate. The palpebral conjunctiva is scraped off of the tarsus with a #15 blade (**Figures 5-9 and 5-10**). This helps create firm adhesions and prevents the formation of epithelial inclusion cysts at the new lateral canthus. The tarsal strip can be shortened at this time if desired (**Figure 5-8**).

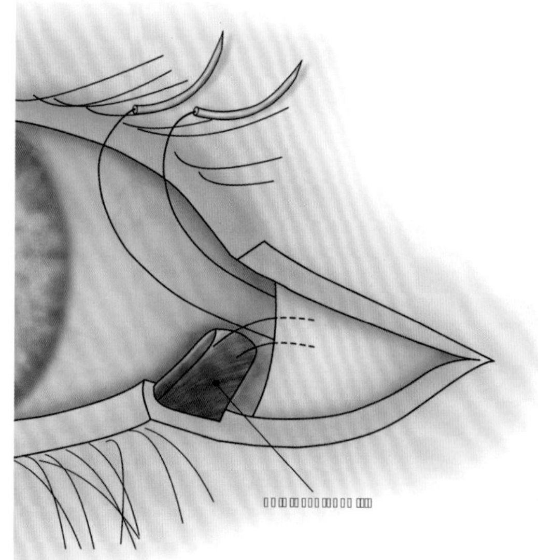

Figure 5-8. Lateral tarsal strip.

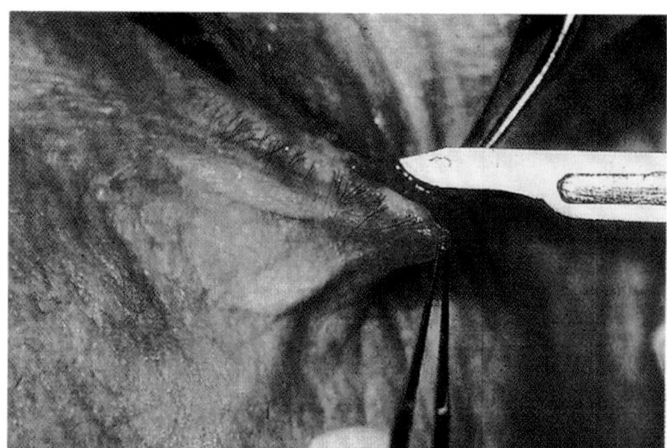

Figure 5-9. Tarsal strip.

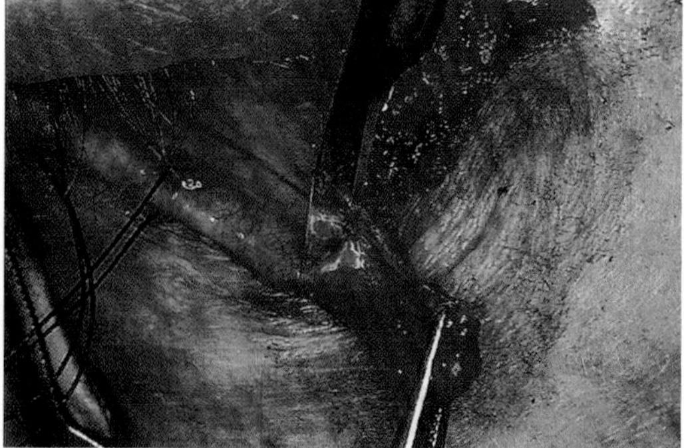

Figure 5-10. Tarsal strip.

Various sutures may be used to reattach the lower lid, including permanent sutures (5-0 undyed nylon is commonly used), or absorbable (we commonly use 5-0 Vicryl on a half-circle needle). The needle is passed through the superior aspect of the tarsal strip under the previously marked point on the lid margin (this will be the new lateral canthal position on the lower lid) in an anterior to posterior direction. The needle is regrasped and passed through the periosteum on the internal aspect of the lateral

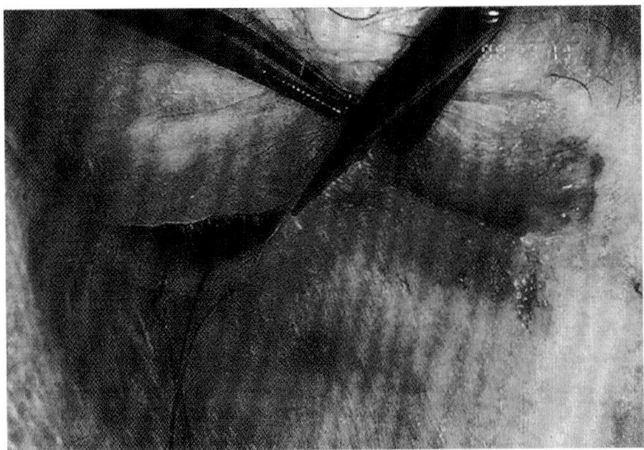

Figure 5-11. Tarsal strip.

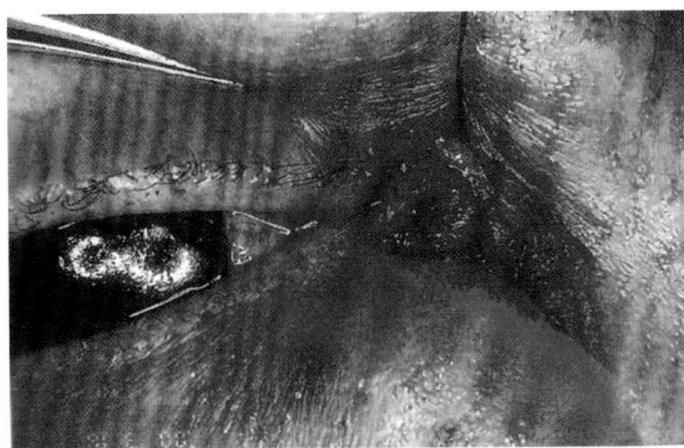

Figure 5-13. Tarsal strip.

orbital rim superior to the lateral canthal tendon insertion, and tied securely. If performed correctly, the surgeon will first encounter bone inside the lateral orbital rim, then "walk" the needle up until it is just able to grasp the periosteum and be brought out through the lateral tissue. A second suture is passed in the same manner through the inferior aspect of the tarsal strip, regrasped, and passed through the periosteum. It is crucial to place the tarsal strip on the internal aspect of the orbital rim to prevent anterior displacement of the lateral canthus. A slight overcorrection in both height and tension is desired intraoperatively (**Figures 5-11–5-13**). An additional 5-0 Vicryl suture can be used to engage the orbicularis from the lateral aspect of the lower lid and tighten it laterally and superiorly and anchored to the deep muscular tissue laterally. The lateral canthal angle is reconstructed with a buried interrupted 5-0 Vicryl Rapide suture (or chromic gut). Skin is closed with interrupted sutures (5-0 or 6-0 Vicryl Rapide, chromic gut, or plain gut). The first skin suture includes a deep muscular bite to avoid webbing in the lateral canthal area

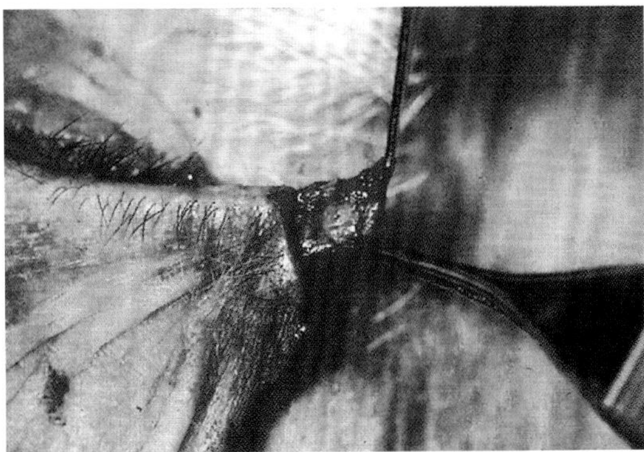

Figure 5-12. Tarsal strip.

Ectropion with Retraction (Vertical Insufficiency)

Evaluation: Frank ectropion or significant laxity on exam (same criteria for #2 above). In addition, vertical insufficiency is present as well (i.e., positive two-finger test).

Surgical Repair

This procedure requires the above lateral tarsal strip with vertical augmentation of the middle/posterior lamella. After the tarsal strip has been fashioned, but before passing any sutures, an incision is made just beneath the inferior tarsus on the palpebral conjunctival (inner) surface of the lower lid. The incision should begin just lateral to the position of the punctum and extend to the lateral surgical incision. Incision is best made with a fine-tipped needle on a cutting cautery unit (or CO_2 laser). Blunt and minimal sharp dissection is performed to fashion a recipient bed between the inferior tarsal border and the conjunctival edge (this may also contain the edge of the lower eyelid retractors—occasionally visible as a white horizontal line 5–10 mm inferior to the cut edge) (**Figure 5-14**).

There are numerous options for a lower eyelid spacer graft. The "gold standard" is an autologous hard palate graft (**Figure 5-15**). More often, a donor graft is used. These are acellular dermal grafts from various sources (currently in use are human, porcine, or fetal bovine). Once the graft is harvested or prepared, it is cut to size. The hard palate can be sized slightly larger than the measured height deficit (i.e., if 2 mm of inferior sclera show preoperatively, size the graft with a maximum vertical height of 3–4 mm). The donor grafts should be sized at least twice as large as the measured vertical deficit.

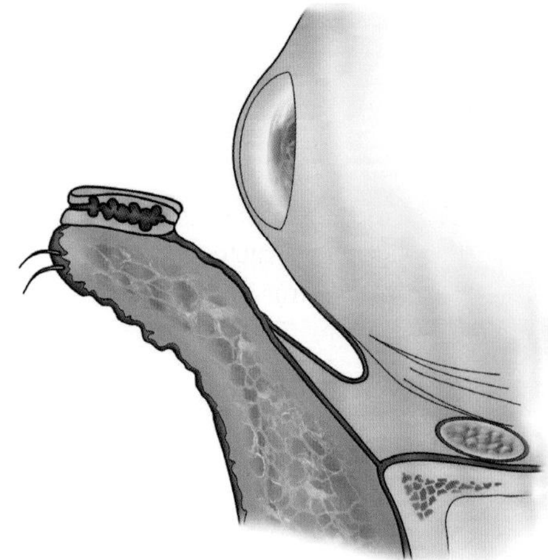

Figure 5-14. Spacer Graft.

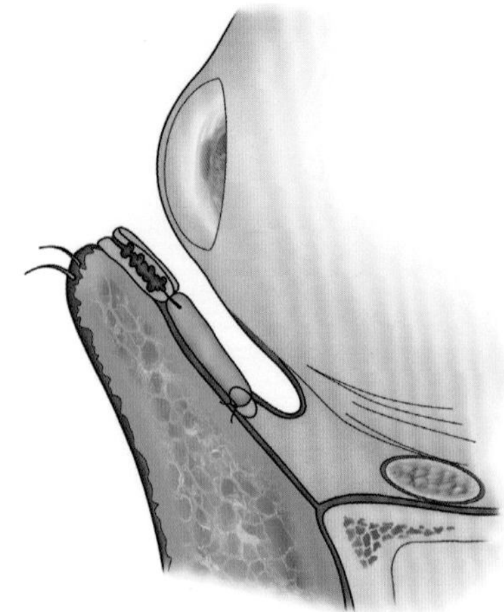

Figure 5-16. Schematic of space graft.

All grafts should be tapered (larger laterally to smaller nasally). The graft is sutured into the recipient bed with a combination of buried interrupted and/or running sutures. Again, the 5-0 Vicryl Rapide suture is our preferred suture, although chromic gut is also an option. If needed, a double-armed chromic gut can also be placed at full thickness through the center of the graft and tied over a bolster on the skin surface to further stabilize the graft position **(Figure 5-16)**.

After the graft is positioned, the tarsal strip is attached and lower-lid blepharoplasty is completed. Obviously, in cases requiring this level of surgical repair, skin should be removed VERY CONSERVATIVELY during simultaneous blepharoplasty (i.e., pinch technique).

Preoperative Cicatricial Ectropion or Retraction

If preoperative assessment reveals a cicatricial ectropion or retraction, lower eyelid blepharoplasty should be deferred until the eyelid malposition is surgically corrected.

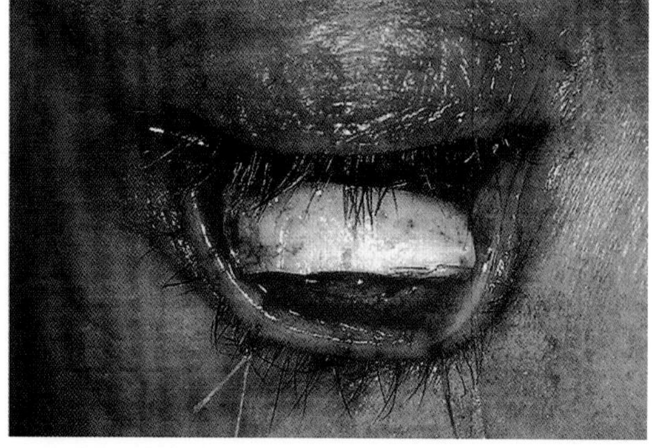

Figure 5-15. Hard palate spacer graft.

Punctal Ectropion

Any punctual eversion present can be corrected by a medial spindle procedure. After local anesthesia, a diamond-shaped excision of conjuntiva and underlying inferior lid retractors is fashioned. This diamond is 4–6 mm high, 6–8 mm long, and located about 4 mm below the punctum. One or two double-armed 5-0 chromic sutures are placed in a buried fashion to reapproximate the edges of the defect, then brought out through the skin and tied over bolster(s). This will rotate the punctum toward the globe **(Figure 5-17)**.

Ectropion and Lower-Lid Retraction Following Blepharoplasty

Lid retraction with or without ectropion is a common and dreaded complication following lower-eyelid blepharoplasty. It is more severe in patients who have also had an upper-eyelid–shortening procedure. Lagophthalmos can lead to exposure keratopathy and persistent irritation. Patients present with scleral show, round "sad-looking" eyes, lateral canthal tendon laxity, photophobia, and tearing. Surgery is done to correct vertical deficiency and horizontal laxity while restoring function and aesthetics without the use of skin grafts. Lower-eyelid retraction following cosmetic surgery is multifaceted. Lid malposition away from the globe may be due to anterior lamella deficiency. Eyelid laxity is usually caused by lateral canthal tendon weakness or disinsertion. Middle lamella inflammation leads to scarring that pulls the lower eyelid down from its normal position (**Figure 5-18**). Inflammation of the orbital fat pads results in fibrosis and shrinkage of the orbital septum anteriorly and the capsulopalpebral fascia posteriorly. These are the tissue planes that envelop the orbital fat. Consequently, dense scarring of the lower-lid retractors and orbital septum prevents the lid from moving vertically to cover the cornea and protect the globe. Furthermore, these signs and symptoms are exacerbated by aging changes such as lower eyelid and midface descent.

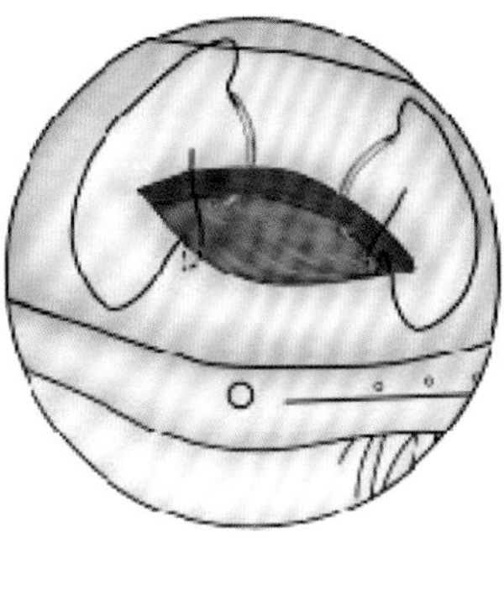

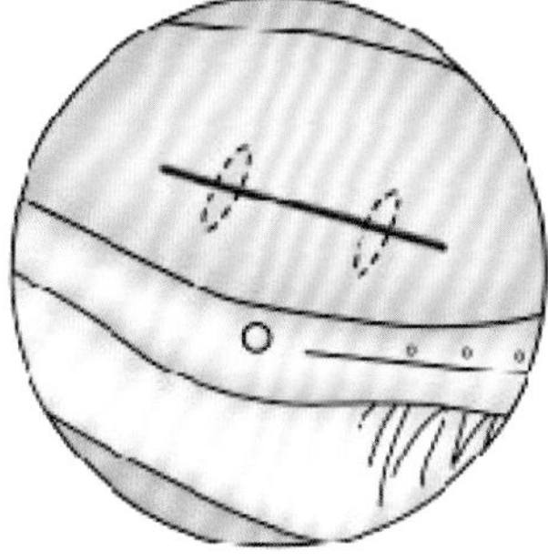

Figure 5-17. Medial spindle.

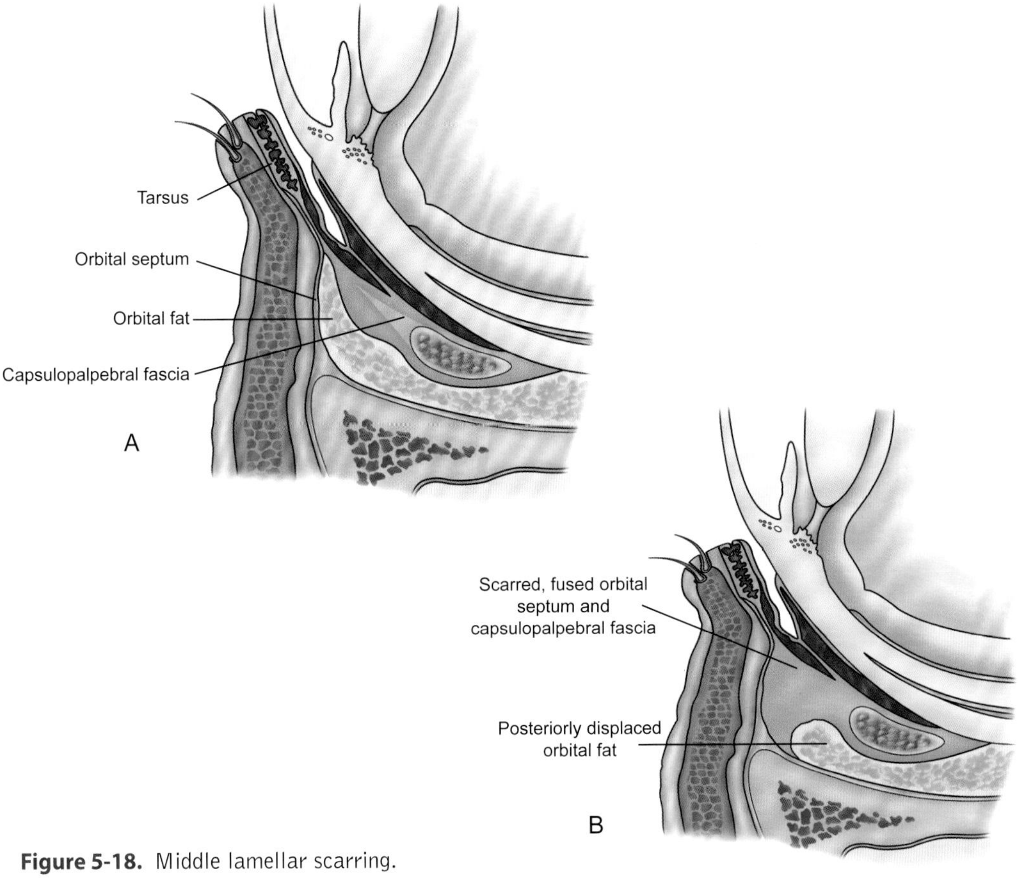

Evaluation

Patients are evaluated to determine which pathologic components of lid retraction are present. First, the lateral canthal angle is pulled down. If the angle is mobile, the lateral canthal tendon is lax. If the lower lid returns to an appropriate position with upward and lateral displacement, then lateral canthal tightening alone is a proper surgical choice (this is rarely the case in the postblepharoplasty setting). If this is truly felt to be a viable surgical plan, a tarsal

Figure 5-18. Middle lamellar scarring.

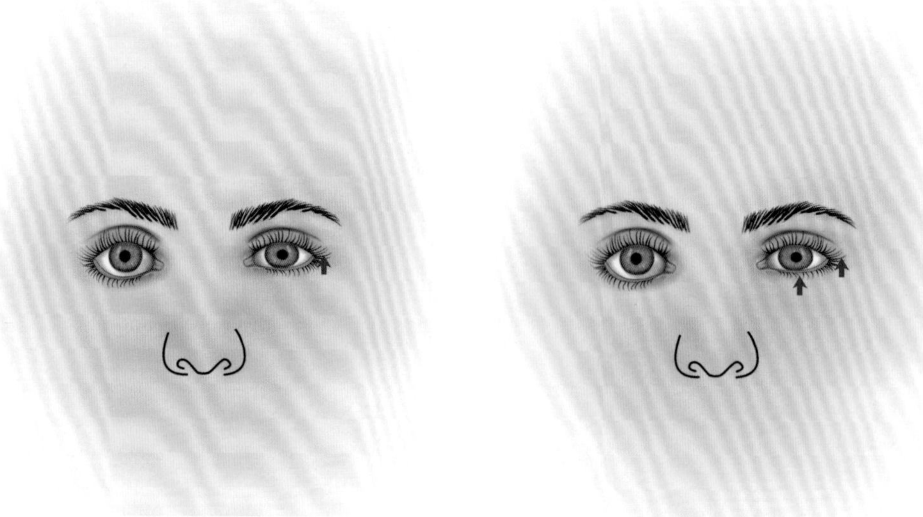

Figure 5-19. Retraction Evaluation.

strip procedure will be performed—this time using a combination of one absorbable and one nonabsorbable suture for canthal fixation. If the central portion of the eyelid fails to reach the inferior limbus, then a spacer graft is necessary to elevate the lower lid along with lateral tightening—as described above (**Figures 5-19 and 5-20**).

If vertical scarring is significant, then subperiosteal midface lifting may prove useful. In severe cases of retraction associated with skin loss, a full-thickness skin graft may be unavoidable (**Figure 5-21; 5-22**).

Surgical Technique

Several techniques have been described to repair lid retraction with lower-lid and midface elevation. The one described here is the author's current method. This procedure is usually performed under general anesthesia, with local injection added for additional pain management and hemostasis.

The procedure begins with harvesting a hard palate mucosa graft. Acellular dermal grafts already mentioned may also be used. Placing this graft releases the middle lamellar scar, recesses the capsulopalpebral fascia, and supports the tarsus in an

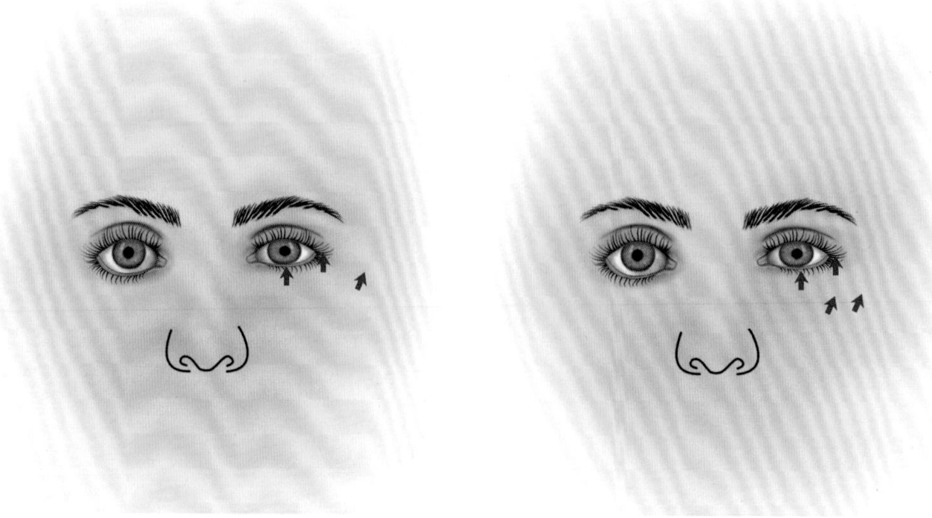

Figure 5-20. Retraction Evaluation.

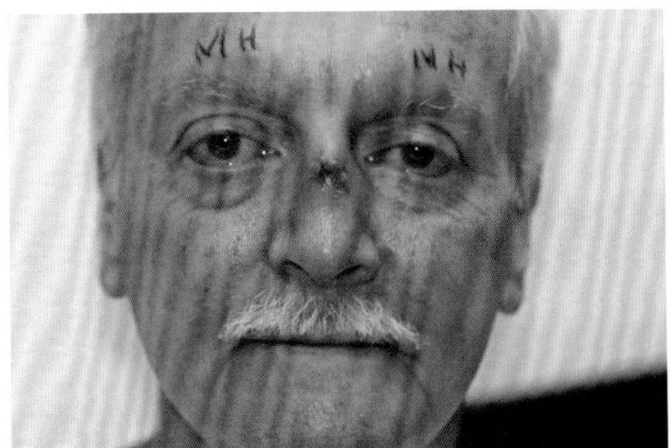

Figure 5-21. Lid retraction.

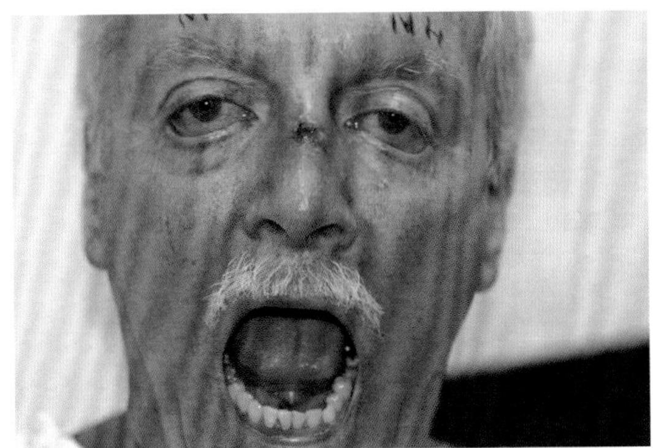

Figure 5-22. Lid retraction with anterior lamella deficiency.

elevated position. If a hard palate graft is planned, patients have a dental plate made prior to surgery to wear postoperatively until the donor site heals. A side-mouth bite block is placed. The graft site is marked and injected with Lidocaine 2% with epinephrine. The donor site is lateral to the midline, just posterior to the alveolar ridge, and 1 to 2 mm anterior to the soft palate to avoid the palatine vessels, which are located at the junction of the hard and soft palates. These grafts are usually 5 mm wide and 20–25 mm long. The mucosa is incised with a no. 11 blade or cutting cautery, carefully leaving the mucoperiosteum intact. It is dissected in a submucosal plane with a crescent blade or periosteal elevator. Hemostasis is achieved with gentle cautery, and the graft is placed in saline-soaked gauze for later use. The donor bed may be packed with gel foam at this time if desired (**Figure 5-23**).

A lateral canthotomy and inferior cantholysis (described previously) are created to permit manipulation of the lower lid. The incision is extended medially through the conjunctiva, separating the lower-lid retractors from the inferior tarsus. Dissection continues inferiorly to release any adhesions and scarring between the capsulopalpebral fascia and orbital septum. Once the lower lid is free, attention is turned to the orbital rim periosteum. This is incised and periosteum is elevated inferiorly

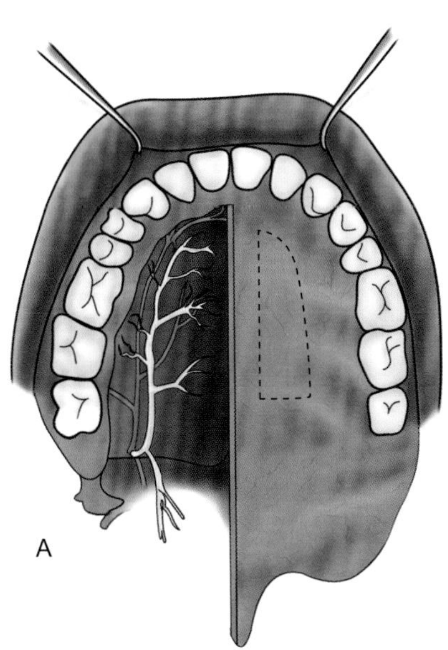

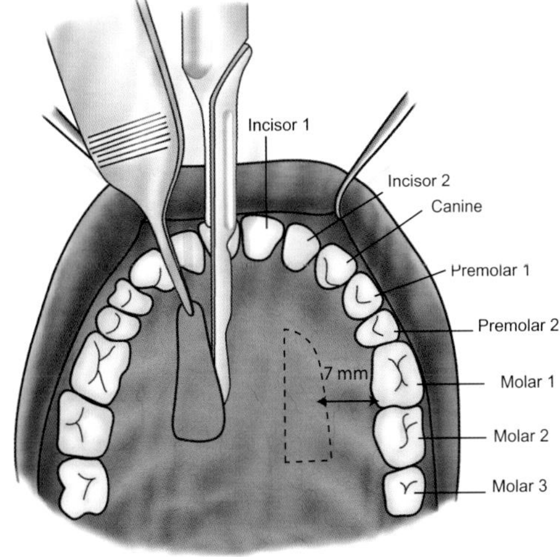

Figure 5-23. Hard palate graft.

until the malar recess is reached. Damage to the infraorbital nerve is avoided medially. To completely release the midface and recruit a maximum amount of tissue for the lower lids, a second dissection site is created in the gingival mucosa. Cautery is used to produce a 1.5–2 cm subperiosteal incision superoateral to the incisor. The periosteum is elevated toward the malar eminence until the prior dissection is reached. At this point, the area from the inferior orbital rim to the nasolabial fold is mobile. Sutures can secure the midface in an elevated position. Currently, however, the authors are using the ENDOTINE Midface B for fixation. The leash end is placed in the gingival incision, guided superiorly, and grasped with a hemostat at the inferior orbital rim. Pressure is applied to the cheek where the fixation platform engages the soft tissue. The leash end is then pulled upward, lifting the cheek and lower lid. Once the desired height is obtained, a hole is made with a handheld drill in the orbital rim. A screw is placed and the residual leash is cut away. If needed, additional support can be obtained laterally with suture fixation.

Focus is brought back to the hard palate mucosa graft. It is thinned of fatty tissue using scissors. A 5-0 Vicryl Rapide or 5-0 chromic suture attaches the graft to the inferior tarsal border and the recessed capsulopalpebral fascia. The knots should be buried. If AlloDerm or other donor material is used, the piece is cut to size and secured in the same fashion. Note that of all the dermal donor material currently available, only AlloDerm has a preferred orientation —with the basement membrane side oriented toward the globe.

Once the midface is elevated and the lower lid is released and lengthened, the lateral canthus must be reconstructed. A tarsal strip is fashioned as previously described. A minimal amount of tarsus, if any, is resected. It is then reattached to the periosteum at the internal portion of the lateral orbital rim as high as possible. Slight overcorrection provides extra support to the eyelid and resolves over time. If needed for better canthal support, two drill holes can be made at the desired position of the new lateral canthus through the bone of the lateral orbital rim (3–5 mm posterior to the rim) and the tarsal strip repositioned using a 4-0 Prolene suture or equivalent.

A frost suture is placed for several days. The dental obturator is positioned in the mouth. A soft diet is recommended for 7 days.

Cicatricial Ectropion

Patients with scarring and shortening of the anterior lamella require a full-thickness skin graft. Common donor sites include the upper eyelid, postauricular skin, or the supraclavicular fossa. If a localized scar is present, a Z-plasty may be performed instead of a graft. These procedures are often coupled with horizontal tightening.

The lid is marked prior to injection at the incision site. In the lower lid, this is 1–2 mm below the lashes. In the upper lid, a mark is made at the desired lid crease. Lidocaine 2% is injected into the affected eyelid as well as the donor site. Both areas are then prepared and draped. A 4-0 silk traction suture through the tarsus at the lid margin places the lid on stretch. A #15 blade is used to make an incision, and sharp dissection is performed to raise a skin flap and release all scar tissue. Once all scaring is released, excellent hemostasis must be maintained to prevent hematoma formation under the graft, as it may compromise its survival. If horizontal laxity is present, a tightening procedure is completed at this time. The size of the recipient bed is now measured. Attention is returned to the donor site. The graft is outlined with a marking pen, and a template may be used to size the graft. It should be slightly larger than the recipient area to allow for shrinkage. The graft is incised and elevated from the subcutaneous tissue using blunt and sharp dissection. The defect is closed in layers. The skin graft is then thinned by placing it skin-side down on the surgeon's finger or on a sterile tray. Westcott scissors are used to excise subcutaneous tissue evenly until the rete papillae are visible. The graft is then sutured into place with 6-0 plain gut sutures (**Figures 5-24–5-26**). Full-thickness slits may be placed

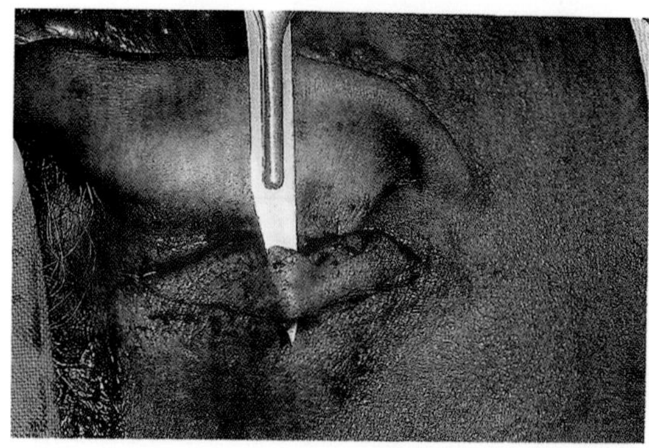

Figure 5-24. Cicatricial ectropion repair.

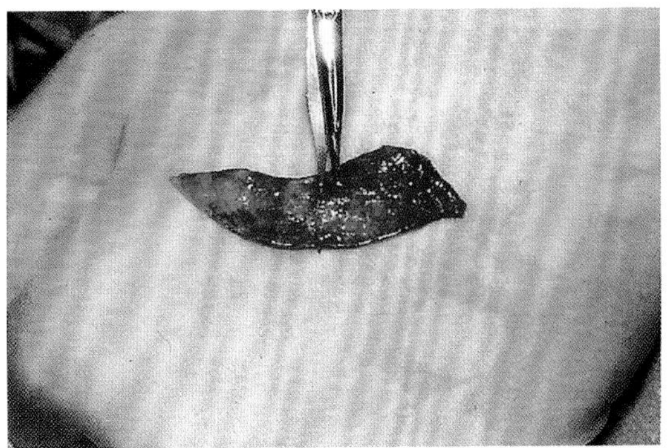

Figure 5-25. Cicatricial ectropion repair.

in the graft to allow fluid to drain. The traction sutures are then taped to the forehead, placing the lid on stretch (**Figure 5-27**). Frost sutures may be used instead. Antibiotic ointment and a Telfa dressing are placed over the graft, and eye patches over the Telfa create a pressure dressing. Aquaplast is molded over the patches. This dressing is left in place for 3–5 days.

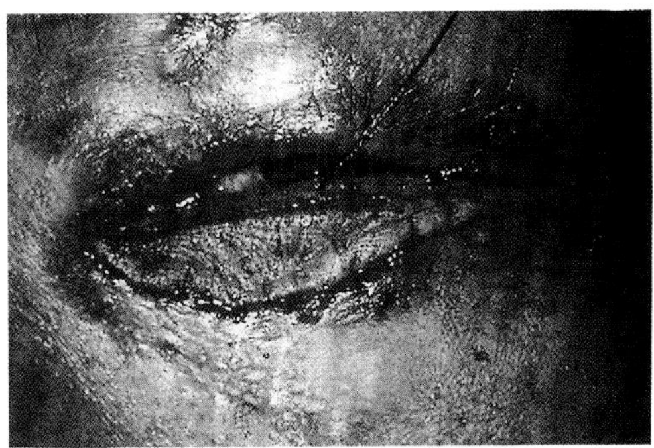

Figure 5-26. Cicatricial ectropion repair.

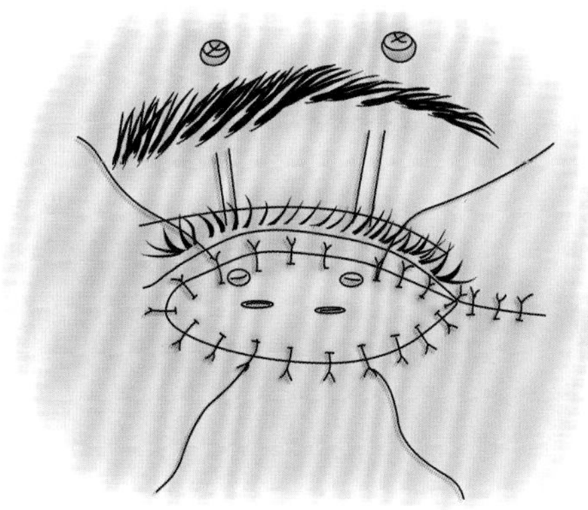

Figure 5-27. Cicatricial ectropion repair schematic.

Suggested Readings

1. Frueh BR, Schoengarth LD. Evaluation and treatment of the patient with ectropion. *Ophthalmology* 89: 1049, 1982.
2. Patipa M. The evaluation and management of lower eyelid retraction following cosmetic surgery. *Plast Reconstr Surg* 106:438, 2000.
3. Hawes MJ, Dortzbach RK. The microscopic anatomy of the lower eyelid retractors. *Arch Ophthalmol* 100:1313, 1318, 1982.
4. Doxanas MT. Eyelid abnormalities: Ectropion, entropion, trichiasis. In: Tasman W, Jaeger EA. eds. Duane's Clinical Ophthalmology. Philadelphia: J.B. Lippincott, 1993.
5. Fagien S. Algorithm for canthoplasty: The lateral retinacular suspension: A simplified suture canthopexy. *Plast Reconstr Surg* 1999;103:2042–2053.
6. Arthurs BP. Ectropion. In: Della Rocca RC, Bedrossian EH, Arthurs BP., eds. Ophthalmic Plastic Surgery Decision Making and Techniques. New York: McGraw-Hill, 2002.
7. Gavaris PT, Kaplan LJ. Management of entropion and ectropion. focal points 1983: Clinical Modules for Ophthalmologists, American Academy of Ophthalmology, module 12.
8. Tse DT, Neff AG. Ectropion In: Chen WP, ed. Oculoplastic Surgery: The Essentials. New York: Thieme, 2001.
9. Nowiski TS, Anderson RL. The medial spindle procedure for medial ectropion. *Arch Ophthalmol* 1985; 103:1750–1753.
10. Jordan DR, Anderson, RL. The lateral tarsal strip revisited. *Arch Ophthalmo*. 107:604, 1989.
11. Patipa M. Transblepharoplasty lower eyelid and midface rejuvenation: Part 1. Avoiding complications by utilizing lessons learned from the treatment of complications. *Plast Reconstr Surg* 113:1459, 2004.
12. Patel BCK, Patipa M, Anderson RL, et al. Management of post blepharoplasty lower eyelid retraction with hard palate grafts and lateral tarsal strip. *Plast Reconstr Surg* 99:1251–1260, 1997.
13. Shorr N, Fallor MK. "Madame Butterfly" procedure: Combined cheek and lateral canthal suspension procedure for post blepharoplasty, "round eye," and lower eyelid retraction. *Ophthalmic Plast Reconstr Surg* 1985;1:229–235.
14. Dortzbach, RK eds. Ophthalmic Plastic Surgery: Prevention and Management of Complications. New York: Raven Press, Ltd., 1994.

6

Asian Blepharoplasty

Samuel M. Lam, MD

Introduction

Asian blepharoplasty is a term that mandates clarification at the outset. In general, Asian blepharoplasty may refer to cosmetic upper and/or lower eyelid surgery for the East Asian patient. However, the term has come to possess a very specific meaning that involves creation of a supratarsal crease in the Asian patient who is born without one. Formerly, "Westernization" was in vogue approximately 25 years ago when the primary objective was to establish a high supratarsal crease and a relatively skeletonized upper-eyelid sulcus in order to emulate the Caucasian, or Occidental, features. However, Westernization is truly an outdated appellation that only serves to ascribe motivational factors for the procedure that are oftentimes not present and, even more so, may carry connotations about the technical aspects of the procedure that are rarely performed today.

This chapter focuses primarily on the narrow definition of supratarsal crease formation, also known in common parlance as the double-eyelid procedure, or double-eyelid blepharoplasty. In addition, this chapter also discusses the cultural, psychological, and technical dimensions of performing upper blepharoplasty in an Asian individual who either was born with a supratarsal crease or had a supratarsal crease formed many years prior and now presents with dermatochalasis that warrants correction. Accordingly, this chapter will resonate even with the aesthetic facial surgeon who never intends to undertake traditional double-eyelid Asian blepharoplasty but may want to manage the aging Asian eyelid that already exhibits a supratarsal crease and the related pearls and pitfalls encountered along the way.

The lower eyelid of the Asian patient has been shown to exhibit anatomic/histologic features that are unique and different from the Caucasian eyelid. These subtle anatomic differences are discussed in the following section but hold very little clinical import for the practicing surgeon. Besides these arcane matters, the differences in overall Asian facial features and how those features relate to blepharoplasty will be elaborated and are important when approaching the prospective Asian patient. A systematic appraisal of the aging Asian eyelid and face will be outlined in order to better understand how to address the eyelids as an aesthetic component of the overall face. As part of this strategy, facial fat contouring, which I use extensively as a principal and adjunctive measure in global facial rejuvenation in both the Asian and non-Asian patient (with different objectives and modification of technique), will be elaborated.

Historically, the very first documented Asian blepharoplasty intended to create a supratarsal crease was reported in 1896 by a Japanese surgeon named Mikamo during the Meiji Restoration. His technique involved using a simple transcutaneous suture ligation. The suture technique has remained popular as an expedient yet beneficial solution to create the supratarsal crease in the Asian patient, especially in Japan. However, reported incidences of eventual fold loosening and loss have restrained the enthusiasm and widespread adoption of this technique elsewhere. Incisional-based techniques range from a limited partial incision to a full incision that spans the distance of the upper eyelid. As many practitioners of the art of Asian blepharoplasty that exist, there are as many variations and modifications in technique. Combination of suture and partial-incision techniques have been reported in the literature as well as extended partial-incision methods that at times still may incorporate various elements of suture ligation.

I have trained in all three major techniques, that is, suture, partial-incision, and full-incision methods. I began my career with the partial-incision method, which I found to be expedient in both its technical execution as well as in the more limited recovery time involved. However, I use the full-incision method almost exclusively today owing to the flexibility in treating both younger and older patients as well as the lower morbidity profile. With a broader expanse of levator-to-skin fixation, all fixation sutures may be removed at the end of the first week without risk of fold loss. However, in more abbreviated incision methods, permanent buried sutures must remain intact in order to limit the risk of fold loss. This assurance is not always encountered, and occasional suture extrusion is not only a nuisance but also potentially problematic engendering potential fold loss. In addition, a shorter incision may be more visible, as there can be a point of visual delineation where the incision starts and stops on the eyelid surface. For these minor (or not so minor) issues, I now perform the full-incision technique only. This chapter focuses on the technical issues of this primary method that employs a full incision for supratarsal-crease creation.

Facial Analysis

The anatomy of the Asian upper eyelid is complex and often debated. The classification of the Asian upper eyelid can be more accurately delineated into those with a discernible eyelid crease, those with a low or partial fold, and those without any fold at all. For all practical matters, the latter two categories can be considered to be one and the same, as a partially visible or a very low crease should be corrected with a standard Asian blepharoplasty technique as if no crease existed at all. The type of eyelid crease that is present is predicated on the height at which the levator aponeurosis inserts into the overlying dermis, which in general is lower than in that of the Caucasian. Alternatively, proponents have argued that the levator itself does not insert at all into the skin but fine fibrous septae that extend from the tarsus into the skin define the fold instead. These academic matters attempt to justify clinical technique at times, whether the levator or tarsus should be suspended to the skin. In my opinion, the underlying anatomy should have little bearing on choice of surgical method. The aesthetic result and morbidity profile of a certain technique should be the only persuading factors for the surgeon in his selection of method.

Besides the absence of a supratarsal crease, the Asian upper eyelid may be characterized by relative fullness in eyelid contour and a narrower palpebral fissure. This condition most likely arises from the absence or low insertion of the levator to skin, which permits the preaponeurotic fat to descend further inferiorly leading to both a fuller eyelid and a narrower palpebral aperture. The relatively low fusion of the orbital septum to the levator aponeurosis has been called the septoaponeurotic sling. Therefore, the fullness of the Asian upper-eyelid contour can be more accurately ascribed to the low position of the levator to skin adhesion than to the abundance of orbital fat. Accordingly, I am very conservative with orbital fat removal in most cases especially considering that with aging ongoing, fat loss will contribute to a skeletonized and aged countenance, which I then correct with an autologous fat transfer. However, an exuberant amount of fat may still be encountered—a condition I have found to be more prevalent in some Korean patients—and should be addressed with proportionate fat reduction.

The epicanthal fold that extends along the medial extent of the upper eyelid is found in 40–90% of Asians to a varying degree. This skin fold descends in an arc to camouflage the caruncle, or lacrimal lake, and may benefit from modification at times. A wide range of options for amelioration of the epicanthal fold has been espoused; however, the majority of them are associated with a high incidence of unfavorable scarring and web formation. Conservative modification of the epicanthus that remains within the skin fold itself, combined with shortening of the medial canthal ligament, has proven to be a reliable technique with limited morbidity.

The superior obliquity of the lateral canthus vis-à-vis the position of the medial canthus has been cited as the reason for the ethnic appearing slant of Asian eyes. Various Z-plasty techniques have been espoused to modify this condition with a high incidence of unfavorable and difficult to correct scarring. In addition, lateral canthoplasty techniques for opening the palpebral aperture wider in a horizontal axis tends to fail to achieve the aesthetic objective owing to eventual reclosure of the canthus. In general, canthal modifications should be reserved for the individual who is cognizant of the limitations of the technique including the associated risks.

Besides the aforementioned anatomic differences in the upper eyelid between the Asian and the Caucasian, a few dissimilarities have been reported in the anatomy of the lower eyelid as well. One cadaveric study discovered very little to no adhesion between the orbital septum and capsulopalpebral fascia at the lower border of the tarsal plate. In a correlative study with magnetic resonance imaging (MRI), the orbital fat in the Asian eyelid was observed to extend more anteriorly vis-à-vis position to the orbital rim. In Asians who did not have a well-defined upper-eyelid crease, the study found that the orbital fat tended to approach the inferior border of the tarsus. No discernible differences were noted in the suborbicularis oculi fat (SOOF) between the Asian and the Caucasian. These anatomic differences in the lower eyelid really remain an academic distinction without significant clinical import.

When approaching the younger Asian patient, the exercise of facial analysis is relatively straightforward. The absence of a supratarsal crease or the presence of a poorly defined and low crease would motivate the individual to seek supratarsal crease formation. Perhaps the most important related anatomic feature when evaluating the patient for Asian blepharoplasty is the nose, more specifically the nasal dorsum. A very low nasal bridge can give the illusion of wider set eyes or accentuate the prominence of the epicanthus. However, engaging in a conversation with a prospective patient about augmentation rhinoplasty who only mentions desire for a double-eyelid procedure may be construed as offensive. Care should be taken when the surgeon evaluates adjacent facial features if the patient is desirous of change of only the stated feature. The impact of rhinoplasty on Asian blepharoplasty in most cases is not significant except in wider set eyes, larger eyes, prominent epicanthal folds, or noses with very shallow radixes. In these cases, it may be worthwhile to explain to the patient the benefit of a related cosmetic rhinoplasty. Discussion of operative techniques for Asian rhinoplasty lies beyond the scope of this chapter. In brief, my preference is to combine expanded polytetraflouroethylene sheets for dorsal augmentation and cartilage tip-plasty maneuvers in most clinical cases.

For the aging Asian eyelid, there are a host of psychological and anatomic issues that must be considered—the details of which are thoroughly discussed in the following section on preoperative considerations. However, for sake of clarity, my overall strategy is outlined in approaching the Asian periorbital region except for the actual Asian blepharoplasty, which will be reserved for the following section. This strategy also applies to the non-Asian eyelid as well (with some modifications that will be clearly stated). There has been an ongoing convergence in our aesthetic appraisal of the aging eyelid across all racial divides. In the past, the Caucasian eyelid was deemed more attractive after browlift and aggressive upper blepharoplasty that included both exuberant fat and skin removal. However, the hollowing of the periorbital region that occurs with aging would benefit from replacement of fat in order to restore the lost frame of the eye rather than overzealous removal of soft tissue. With this perspective in mind, my preference is to perform conservative skin-only upper blepharoplasty and transconjunctival lower blepharoplasty combined with autologous fat transfer to attain the most ideal aesthetic results. However, the foremost goal in periorbital rejuvenation is not excisional in nature but preservation and restoration of the hollowing frame of the eye. Therefore, a skeletonized and high upper-eyelid crease sulcus that followed the old-style Westernization procedure may not only appear unfavorable in the Asian patient but potentially unaesthetic in the Caucasian individual as well.

Many Asians exhibit a brachycephalic (wider, flatter) face compared with the Occidental dolichocephalic (longer anterior-posterior dimension) face. In particular, the lateral bony cheek and jawl ine can be significantly flared and protuberant in the Korean patient—which can serve to increase the visual width and flattening of the face. The malar region can be considered an extended frame to the eyelid, which should be restored volumetrically with autologous fat transfer at the same time as the eyelid in most cases. To deemphasize the width of the lateral cheek and jawline, the anterior cheek and mentum with fat grafting is accentuated to create a more balanced anterior view and profile for the Asian patient. Sculpting the face in this manner can oftentimes not only improve the overall facial features but also specifically create a more balanced and rejuvenated eyelid appearance.

Preoperative Considerations

As alluded to previously, the approach to the Asian patient can be most easily divided into the younger and older Asian patient. The younger patient is simply desirous of creating a supratarsal crease. However, the older patient may be trying to rejuvenate the aging eyelid with or without reference to creation of a supratarsal crease. In order to understand the pearls and pitfalls of approaching the aging Asian eyelid, that section is divided into three principal categories: the aging Asian eyelid without a crease, the aging Asian eyelid with a natural crease, and the aging Asian eyelid with a previous surgically created crease.

The Younger Asian Eyelid

As mentioned before, the younger patient seeking Asian blepharoplasty is principally desirous of supratarsal crease formation. As dermatochalasis, fat loss, pseudoherniation of fat, wrinkles, dyschromias, and the like are not usually factors; the consultation process is a bit more straightforward. Often, the younger Asian patient brings an exemplar of photographs of celebrities and models who have an eyelid shape that he or she desires. If the Asian patient brings in examples of other Asian models, then dialogue can be fruitful. However, at times, the Asian may bring in Western models, and the surgeon should be careful to understand whether the patient desires Asian blepharoplasty or a more radical alteration in identity that is unachievable with blepharoplasty alone (or with any other surgical modality for that matter). Even when Asians bring in photographs of Asian models, the surgeon should take care to inquire whether the prospective patient likes the photograph for the beauty of the Asian face or the design and shape of the eyelid crease only. This is an important distinction. During my PowerPoint presentation that show numerous examples of my before and after photographs, I begin with examples of different Asian models who have the same eyelid configuration but different facial features. I then ask the prospective patient which eyelid he or she likes better. I try to emphasize that the eyelid crease shape and size are practically identical, but the more attractive facial feature has influenced the prospective patient's opinion. Accordingly, reviewing model's photographs may not always be the most instructive exercise but it does provide a good starting point for discussion.

Generally speaking, I try to understand the prospective patient's desired crease height as the most important aesthetic consideration followed by shape of the eyelid crease. Nowadays, almost all individuals seeking Asian blepharoplasty desire a very narrow eyelid crease height of 1–2 mm above the ciliary margin, as viewed with the eyelid open and

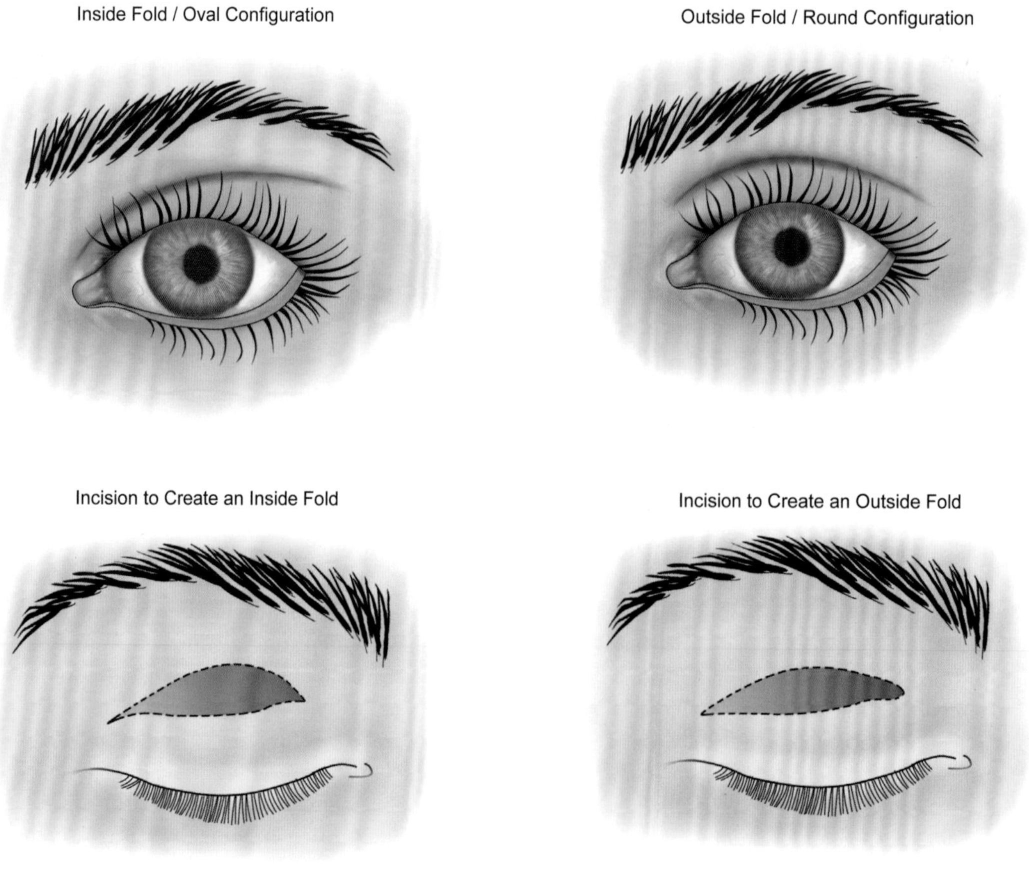

Figure 6-1. Description of variations in eyelid shape showing an inside fold, outside fold, oval configuration, and round configuration as well as how to create an inside versus and outside fold.

staring forward (the surgical marking on the eyelid to achieve this low crease is actually higher and is discussed in the following operative technique section). The eyelid shape refers to two important variables: first, whether the crease terminates within the epicanthus (the so-called "inside fold") or falls medial to the epicanthus (an "open fold"); second, whether the eyelid crease continues across the eyelid at the same height throughout (a "round configuration") or progressively becomes higher toward the lateral aspect (an "oval configuration"). In general, the closed nature of an inside fold is better suited to the flared oval shape eyelid, whereas a fold that remains open medially looks better with a round eyelid configuration **(Figure 6-1)**. The details of how to design skin markings that will result in closed, open, round, and oval shapes are discussed in the section dedicated to operative technique.

Although women may look natural and attractive with a low supratarsal crease (1–2 mm) or, alternatively, a medium-sized crease (3–4 mm), men generally are really candidates for a low supratarsal crease only. A medium or large crease in a male creates both an unnatural and an unsightly feminized appearance. This feminized appearance is evident in men of all races who have undergone an aggressive browlift and/or upper blepharoplasty. Even if the end result of the procedure leaves almost no discernible crease for the male patient, this outcome should be explained to the patient as a favorable one. It is important to explain this possible desired result beforehand, as a comment before a procedure is deemed an explanation and one that follows a procedure is merely an excuse. The reason why supratarsal crease fixation is still a desirable procedure in a male when the outcome may show a negligible or nonexistent crease is the resulting improvement that the procedure affords in opening the palpebral aperture as well as reduction in the perceived fullness of the Asian upper eyelid. Accordingly, it is paramount that a male deciding to undergo Asian blepharoplasty should only concentrate on Asian male models or before and after photographs of other Asian males—unless, of course, the examples are of females who have very low supratarsal creases.

The younger Asian patient desirous of supratarsal crease formation poses the question what is the youngest age acceptable to undertake Asian blepharoplasty in a prospective candidate? This question is particularly relevant, as most Asian patients who present for double-eyelid blepharoplasty are often teenagers. What I look for more than any other factor is psychological, not physical, maturity. Whereas septorhinoplasty in the early teenage years may stunt the growth of the nose, especially in the Asian already wishing for augmentation, Asian blepharoplasty has little effect on overall eyelid changes over the ensuing years. However, a 13-year-old girl who comes to consultation with the mother speaking largely on her behalf is not a good candidate compared with a girl the same age who is more outspoken and whose mother only chimes in for supportive words or queries. Like all aesthetic surgery, understanding the psychological motivation and maturity lies at the heart of determining the likelihood of success and the appropriateness of the undertaking.

During the initial consultation, the surgeon should also evaluate the eyelids for anatomic features that may prove to encumber attaining an excellent aesthetic outcome. As the most often encountered complication that follows Asian blepharoplasty is asymmetry between the two surgically created creases, preoperative asymmetry must be noted, photographed, and explained to the patient. Most oftentimes, preexisting asymmetry is caused by the presence of a poor to nonexistent crease on one side and a more defined crease on the other side. Besides the differences in crease heights, the eyelid that does not bear a well-defined crease often has a concomitantly narrow palpebral aperture as well. Generally, adhering to symmetrical crease creation on both sides can lead to a symmetrical outcome despite the preexisting asymmetry. However, subtle variations in anatomy, especially in levator function, can result in persistence of the asymmetry. These factors should always be enumerated in detail during the preoperative consultation with the prospective patient.

The Aging Asian Eyelid

The Aging Asian Eyelid without a Crease

The aging Asian eyelid without a crease may appear as a simple entity to address. However, there are many nuances that must be elaborated and understood before approaching the aging creaseless Asian eyelid. First, creating a supratarsal crease late in life may alter an individual's perceived self-identity. This unforeseen complication can prove particularly vexing for the male patient, who may have a harder time adjusting to a change in identity than the female patient. As documented with rhinoplasty late in life, men have a more difficult time adjusting to a change in their facial features, especially when that change involves not just rejuvenation but alteration in their appearance to a look they never had in their lifetime. Another factor that compounds this result is the prolonged recovery time involved with the full-incision method, which leaves an individual looking unnatural for several weeks to months. During this time, many women can look more natural than men early on since the higher eyelid crease that results from temporary edema does not look as unnatural on the female. Furthermore, the edematous appearance of the upper eyelid crease can be partially camouflaged with mascara and other makeup products. This option is not readily available to men. For these reasons, counseling an older man who desires double-eyelid procedure must not be taken lightly. Obviously, these concerns should also be thoroughly discussed with the younger male candidate.

Understanding precisely the motivation of a mature Asian patient for blepharoplasty must initiate any aesthetic consultation. Many Asian patients simply desire a rejuvenated appearance but do not necessarily want a supratarsal crease or in fact adamantly refuse to have a supratarsal crease. This scenario is perhaps one of the most difficult to deal with. The surgeon may envision two seemingly favorable options: remove only some extra skin somewhere arbitrarily along the upper eyelid skin (as there is no crease to guide incision placement) with or without removing some of the preaponeurotic adipose tissue that is contributing to the fuller eyelid contour without actually tacking the levator to the skin during the procedure. Both of these solutions can prove to be problematic. Removal of skin only along an arbitrary skin height can lead to a visible scar, as no crease forms afterward to camouflage the incision line. Furthermore, the result is perceived as only minimally beneficial, as the narrow palpebral aperture and full-eyelid contour have not been improved (even though the patient has always had a narrow aperture and full-eyelid contour, these facts simply do not matter). I encountered one patient who had her incision placed less than a millimeter above the ciliary margin to camouflage the incision line. However, the end result was that the patient was dissatisfied and the fullness of the eyelid that ended just above the ciliary margin made the result appear unnatural. If the surgeon elects to remove some adipose tissue postseptally without creating a durable adhesion between the levator and skin, variable (incomplete to complete) crease formation may arise simply due to the inadvertent adhesion from the postseptal tissues to the skin. Personal communication with colleagues has revealed that I am not alone in witnessing this unfavorable result. At times, if the problem is in fact perceived dermatochalasis and, in fact, hollowing of the upper-eyelid sulcus, autologous fat transfer without skin removal may be the best option for the patient.

The Aging Asian Eyelid with a Natural Crease

The aging Asian eyelid with a natural crease may appear to be the simplest variation to address and rightfully so. However, some subtleties regarding patient psychology should be elaborated to ensure a favorable aesthetic outcome as perceived by both the surgeon and patient alike. Because supratarsal fixation is not needed and is not even an issue, Asian blepharoplasty defined as a double-eyelid procedure is not relevant here. However, the Asian patient may still be desirous of eyelid rejuvenation. At first glance, this type of Asian patient who has a natural crease would appear to be like any Caucasian or Occidental patient who desires some removal of upper-eyelid skin redundancy. Even though technical execution of removing skin with or without fat is identical to that of the Occidental counterpart, some cultural issues must be underscored. First and foremost, the Asian patient has a perception of what constitutes a natural-looking Asian eyelid. That perception falls squarely on crease height. If the surgeon simply removes significant upper-eyelid skin, he or she can inadvertently raise the crease height unacceptably. Even a change of 2–3 mm may be verboten. If the surgeon reviews his or her own results for Caucasian patients following upper blepharoplasty, the surgeon may see that the crease height is raised in many of them. Although this higher crease height may go unnoticed by the Western patient, it is glaringly obvious to the Asian patient. Accordingly, I do not remove very much upper-eyelid skin in the aging Asian patient with a natural crease (2–4 mm at most) and only do so with proper consultation and evaluation that the crease is already partially obscured by dermatochalasis. If the crease is high and well defined, I will most likely not attempt any upper-eyelid skin removal at all. A concurrent browlift can further elevate the upper-eyelid crease especially when combined with upper eyelid skin-removal blepharoplasty. Once the crease is elevated, it is almost impossible to lower the crease except for one technique, autologous fat transfer. In the individual with a well-defined upper-eyelid crease, upper-eyelid fullness is generally not a concern. In fact, the upper eyelid ages just as the Caucasian upper eyelid does, that is, with tissue deflation, brow descent, and skin redundancy. Accordingly,

I may elevate the upper eyelid crease somewhat with skin-removal blepharoplasty but would concurrently lower the crease by filling the brow and upper eyelid hollow with fat grafting to yield a more youthful appearance and maintain a favorably low crease height simultaneously.

The Aging Asian Eyelid with a Previous Surgically Created Crease

The aging Asian eyelid that has a previous surgically created crease presents a unique challenge. If the crease was created with a standard full-incision method and was always low and natural appearing, then the patient can be approached just like an Asian individual with a natural crease. Unfortunately, many of the creases that were created 20 years ago or more were truly Westernization procedures, characterized by a high crease and a deep upper-eyelid sulcus. Over time, these creases may have descended to a naturally low height owing to brow descent, upper-eyelid dermatochalasis, and soft-tissue involution. If the patient is asked, he or she may recall that at one time the crease looked very unnatural but that over time the crease progressively assumed a more natural position as it descended. A way to determine how high the crease was in the past is to lift up the redundant upper-eyelid skin and inspect how high the crease was created in the past. Also, a patient that had a high crease formed in the past may still look somewhat unnatural to the casual observer who has difficulty knowing why that is the case. The reason for this look is that the thicker brow skin comes to rest over the eyelid leaving a thickened, unnatural appearance to the upper eyelid.

The main concern when approaching the aging Asian eyelid with a previous surgically created supratarsal crease is unmasking the unnatural, Westernized-appearing eyelid through browlifting and/or upper-eyelid skin removal. Accordingly, judicious skin removal (if any) combined with fat grafting (as needed) may be a more conservative course of action that can limit the risk of exposing a bad prior result.

Technique

Although I developed the philosophy espoused in this chapter, I offer my deepest regard to the technique of full-incision double-eyelid creation to my mentor, John A. McCurdy, Jr., who was kind enough to teach me the method that he has refined over the years. I have made some minor modifications, which I accept full responsibility for any faults and give credit to him for any of the favorable attributes of the technique.

Marking the Eyelid

The first order of business is to confirm with the patient the size and shape of the proposed eyelid crease. The eyelid size can be divided into a small, medium, and large crease. Ninety percent of my patients toda y who desire a supratarsal crease favor a small crease height, which is the most natural eyelid configuration for the Asian. A slightly Westernized look can be attained when creating a medium-sized crease. This variation actually still can be discovered naturally in many Asian individuals. The traditional Westernized, high and sculpted crease is attained with a large crease marking. This technique has almost been entirely relegated to historical interest. I personally do not even perform this type of eyelid crease even if the patient desires to have it, as I do not like the aesthetic result of this unnatural appearing surgery, which I find to be disfiguring.

To mark the eyelid crease, the patient should be in a supine position with his or her eyes gently closed. With the nondominant index finger, the eyelid skin is retracted superiorly until the eyelashes begin to evert to a perpendicular orientation. With the skin held taut in this position, a fine gentian violet marking pen is used to mark an initial point in the center of the eyelid measured with Castroviejo calipers (**Figure 6-2**). For a small crease, the point is placed 6–7 mm above the ciliary margin. For a medium crease, the point is placed 8 mm above the ciliary margin. For a large crease, the point is placed

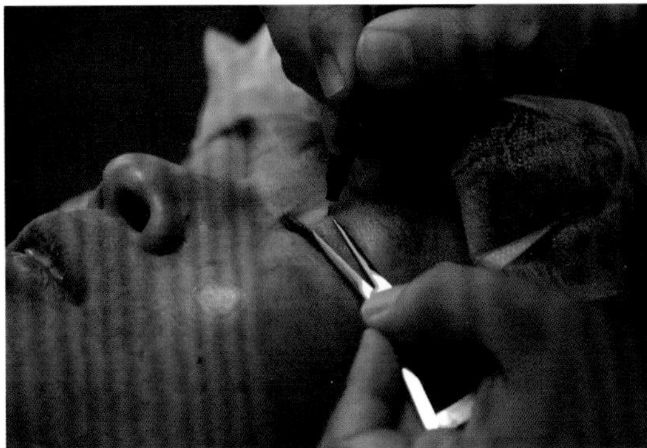

Figure 6-2. To mark the eyelid crease, patient is placed in a supine position and eyelid skin is retracted with the nondominant hand until the eyelashes begin to evert. A fine-tipped gentian violet marking pen is used to mark a point at midpupil at the appropriate height as measured by Castroviejo calipers.

TABLE 6.1 Markings Necessary to Create a Small, Medium, and Large Crease Fold

Size of Crease	*Distance from Ciliary Margin (inferior incision)*	*Amount of Skin Excised*
Small	6–7 mm	3 mm
Medium	8 mm	50% of maxi mum amount of skin removed
Large	9–10 mm	Maximum amount of skin removed minus 3 mm

Second column denotes the distance that the inferior limb of the incision needs to be from the ciliary margin, as marked when the eyelid is under tension/stretch to the point that the eyelashes are everted to a perpendicular orientation. Third column denotes the amount of skin that requires removal (i.e., the marking for the superior limb of the skin incision). For a small crease, only 3 mm of skin needs to be removed. For a medium- and large-sized crease, the "maximum amount of skin removed" refers to the amount of skin that can be pinched with forceps when the patient's eyes are closed without actually causing the eye to open.

9–10 mm above the ciliary margin. The reader is referred to Table 6-1 for a systematic presentation of the requisite measurements for the intended outcome of the desired crease height. With the skin still held taut, the inferior limb is drawn out parallel to the ciliary margin for an oval-shaped eyelid crease and curving about 1 or 2 mm inferiorly from the lateral limbus to lateral canthus for a round eyelid configuration. The medial aspect of the eyelid crease is gently sloped inferiorly just medial to the medial canthus for an inside fold and to the skin dimple that rests medial to the medial canthus for an outside fold. With the skin taut, the upper limb of the skin incision is marked out with caliper and forceps measurements, as prescribed in Table 6-1. The upper and lower limbs are joined laterally with an upward extension of the inferior limb to join the upper limb. The medial extent of the upper limb arcs downward to meet the downward slope of the medial end of the inferior limb.

Both eyelid markings are observed for symmetry with the patient's eyes opened and closed and with the skin held taut and relaxed before continuing (**Figure 6-3**). With symmetry confirmed, the procedure can begin. Although the procedure can be carried out under straight local anesthesia, I have evolved now to incorporate light intravenous sedation, which adds a level of patient comfort that is unsurpassed. Unfortunately, intravenous sedation requires a dedicated sedation/anesthesia provider and a safe, accredited environment based on state regulations. Accordingly, sedation may be a cost-prohibitive venture for such a small procedure as Asian blepharoplasty if the physician does not have his or her own accredited facility. The patient is premedicated the night prior with 0.5 mg of alprazolam oral and 2 hours prior to arrival at the surgery center with the same medication to reduce anxiety. For sedation, I use 2–4 mg of midazalam intravenous push with 0.5 mg increments every 5 minutes based on patient necessity. Intravenous midazolam is combined with 25 to 50 mcg of intravenous sufentanyl to optimize patient comfort. Diprivan 15 mg/kg is administered as a bolus during the procedure based on patient comfort. Generally, it takes me approximately 20–25 minutes to complete the initial portion of dissection from injection of local anesthesia to identification and exposure of the

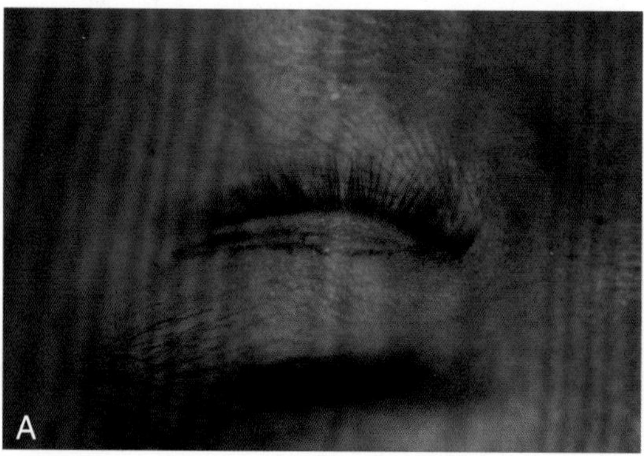

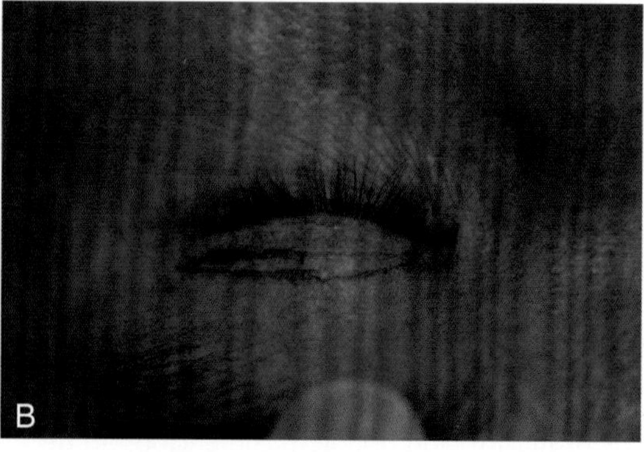

Figure 6-3. (A) Left upper eyelid shown with skin markings in a relaxed state. (B) Same eyelid and skin markings shown with the skin retracted. Note that patient is shown with a small crease marking 7 mm above the ciliary margin with 3 mm of skin marked for removal. Design reveals a round eyelid configuration and a closed inside fold.

levator complex. During this time, it is ideal for the patient to be sedated. However, after this time, the patient should be fully awake to cooperate with eye opening to assess symmetry during placement of levator fixation sutures. Fortunately, the intravenous mixture described above persists for almost the exact time that it requires me to undertake this initial dissection, and the patient is fully cooperative when I need him or her to be.

After the patient is properly sedated, I inject 1 cc of a 50/50 mixture of 1% lidocaine with 1:100,000 epinephrine and 0.25% bupivacaine with 1:200,000 epinephrine along each eyelid incision. I use a 30-gauge needle and raise a subcutaneous wheal, progressing along the entire distance of each eyelid ensuring that a uniform distribution of anesthetic is placed (**Figure 6-4**). By avoiding using linear threading, the likelihood of hematoma formation is greatly reduced. If any bleeding points are noted during injection, immediate and sustained pressure with a 4 × 4 gauze should be applied to avoid a hematoma, which can obscure one's ability to gauge symmetry. After injecting a cubic centimeter of local anesthesia into each eyelid as described, the physician can pinch the incision line along the entire length to ensure a consistent distribution. Povidone–iodine solution is applied delicately to each incision line, upper eyelid, and periorbital region; and the patient is then prepared and draped in the usual sterile fashion.

After 10 minutes, the surgeon can begin to incise the marked incision lines with a no. 15 Bard–Parker surgical blade. The assistant should apply gentle countertraction to the upper eyelid to maintain stability and tension during the incision. The depth of the incision should be just to the level of the orbicularis oculi muscle but not entirely through it because usually several transverse arcades of vessels can begin to be apparent that run in a superior and inferior direction (**Figure 6-5**). As the overlying soft tissue is thinned with the no. 15 blade and the vessels are approached, a bipolar cautery is used to prevent unnecessary hemorrhage with the tips of the cautery erring toward the side of the elliptical skin island that will be discarded. The depth of the incision is then carried the remaining distance through the orbicularis–oculi fibers until the underlying orbital septum is exposed. At this point, the skin island that is situated between the upper and lower limbs of the incision can be removed with fine, microserrated Iris scissors and discarded. Any additional hemostasis can be achieved with bipolar cautery.

With gentle countertraction, a 1–2-mm strip of orbital septum and remaining fibers of the orbicularis oculi are excised with scissors along the entire length of the incision (**Figure 6-6**). The assistant then palpates the eyeball by applying digital pressure above and below the incision line to force the postseptal/preaponeurotic adipose to bulge forward. With the bulge and yellowish hue of preseptal fat visible through the remaining fibers of the orbital septum, a small fenestration through the orbital septum is made with Iris scissors until the yellow fat herniates through the created defect (**Figure 6-7**). With a fine curved hemostat, the tines are passed

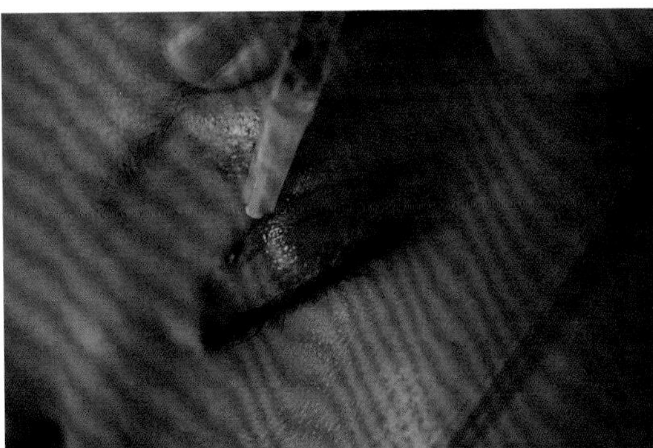

Figure 6-4. Infiltration of local anesthesia with a 50:50 mixture of 1% lidocaine with 1:100,000 epinephrine and 0.25% bupivacaine with 1:200,000 epinephrine. A total of 1 cc of local anesthesia is infiltrated into each eyelid with a 30-gauge needle so that multiple skin wheals are raised rather than in a linear threading technique that could otherwise cause unwanted formation of a hematoma.

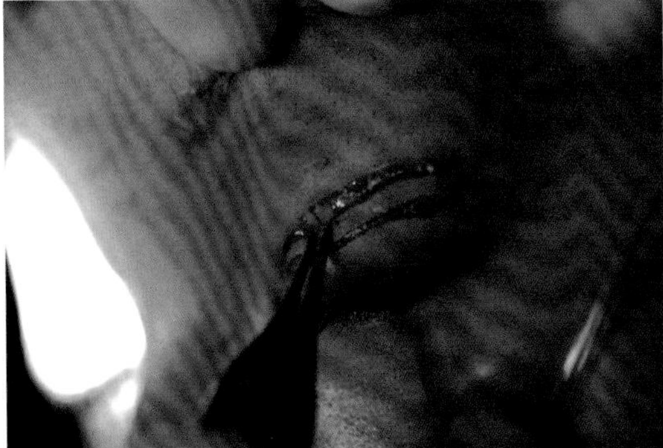

Figure 6-5. After skin has been incised with a no. 15 Bard–Parker blade, some residual fibers of orbicularis oculi are left intact so that the transverse arcade of vessels are not entirely transected, which are then cauterized with a bipolar cautery before continuing.

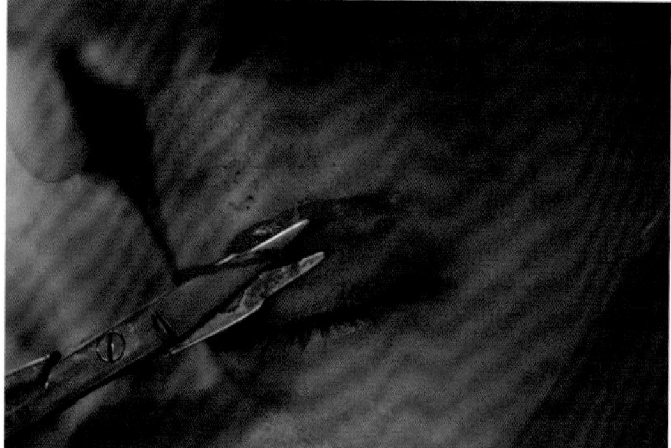

Figure 6-6. After skin island has been discarded, a thin strip of orbital septum and remaining orbicularis oculi fibers are removed with microserrated scissors to expose the underlying orbital fat.

through the defect in a medial direction and, with a gentle spreading action, the orbital septum is lifted up and away from the white levator that remains below (**Figure 6-8**). A bipolar cautery is used to cauterize the orbital septum prior to cutting through it with Iris scissors until the remaining distance of orbital septum is entirely opened up to reveal the levator aponeurosis below (**Figure 6-9**). The orbital fat is teased away with a cotton-tipped applicator to expose the levator fully. At times, the posterior leaf of the orbital septum may appear adherent to the levator complex, which my colleague Young-Kyoon Kim has referred to as the pseudolevator (**Figure 6-10**). These thin, transparent fibers should be elevated and dissected delicately away from the levator complex without damaging the levator to permit improved exposure and fixation of the levator complex.

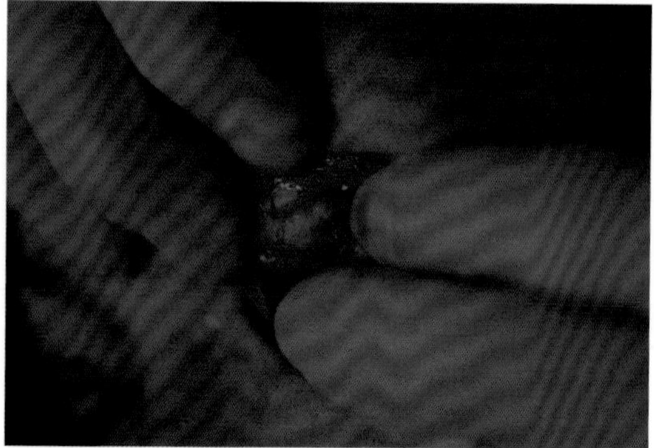

Figure 6-7. With the assistant balloting the eyeball on either side of the incision to propulse the fat pad forward, the surgeon creates a small fenestration through the remaining fibers of the orbital septum to expose fully the underlying orbital fat pad.

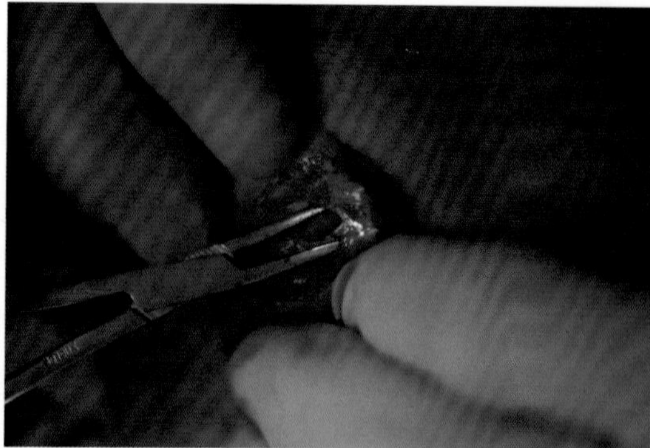

Figure 6-8. With fine curved hemostat, the tines are passed through the defect in a medial direction and with gentle spreading action the orbital septum is lifted up and away from the white levator that remains below.

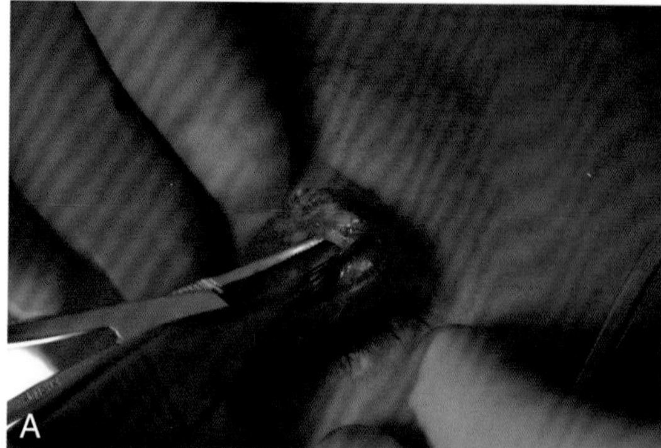

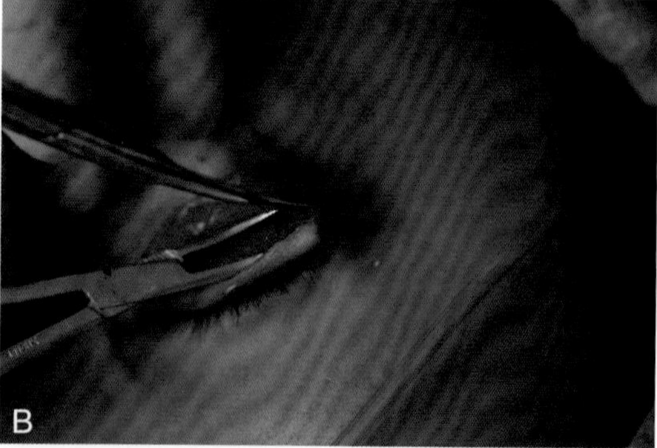

Figure 6-9. (A) Bipolar cautery is used to cauterize the orbital septum (B) prior to cutting through it with Iris scissors until the remaining distance of orbital septum is entirely opened up to reveal the levator aponeurosis below.

The same dissection should be undertaken in the contralateral side until the levator and preaponeurotic fat pads are fully exposed. At this point, any excessive fat that extends beyond a 1-cm cuff under a hemostat clamp should be cut away and cauterized

Figure 6-10. After the orbital fat is fully exposed, a thin wispy layer may be encountered that divides the fat from the levator aponeurosis. This layer tented up in the photograph by fine hemostats represents the posterior leaf of the orbital septum (also termed the pseduolevator) and should be divided to reveal the levator aponeurosis in an unobstructed fashion.

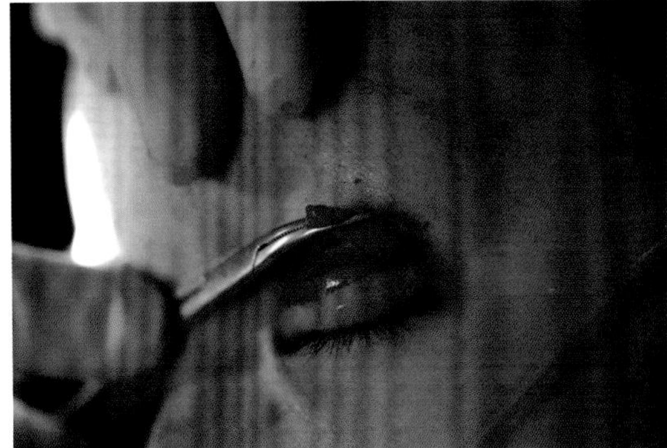

Figure 6-11. Leaving a 1-cm cuff of orbital fat in situ, any excess adipose beyond that measurement can be clamped, cauterized, and removed. Note the levator aponeurosis that resides deep to the fat pad.

(**Figure 6-11**). Remember that the amount of fat that remains should be symmetrical and not the amount of fat that is removed necessarily. Generally speaking, I have progressively become more conservative with adipose removal, as I am an avowed proponent of autologous fat transfer. In the older patient, I will invariably not remove any adipose tissue but instead transfer fat back into the superior orbital rim immediately following Asian blepharoplasty as needed. With the patient adequately sedated, no additional anesthesia is necessary during removal of adipose tissue. However, with straight local anesthesia, 2% of plain lidocaine can be instilled into the portion of the fat pad intended removal to reduce discomfort. The surgeon should be cognizant that no lidocaine can drip onto the levator, which could inadvertently anesthetize the levator function and impair one's ability to gauge overall symmetry. If any lidocaine

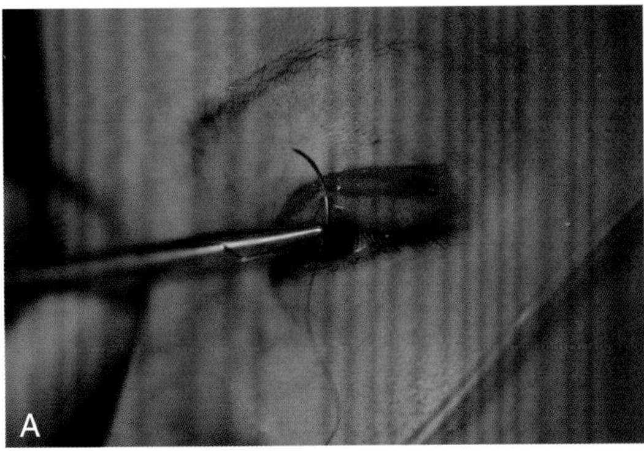

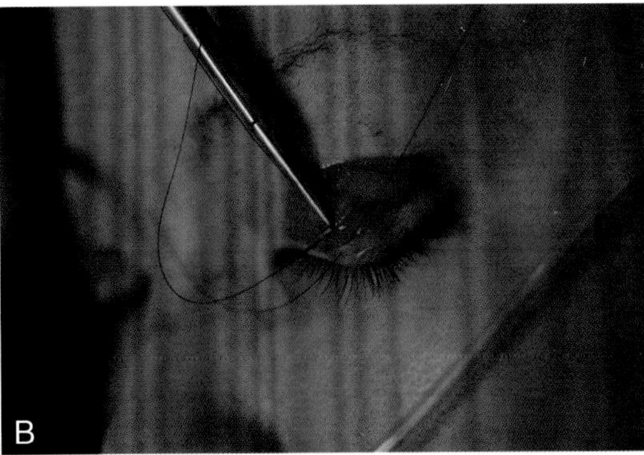

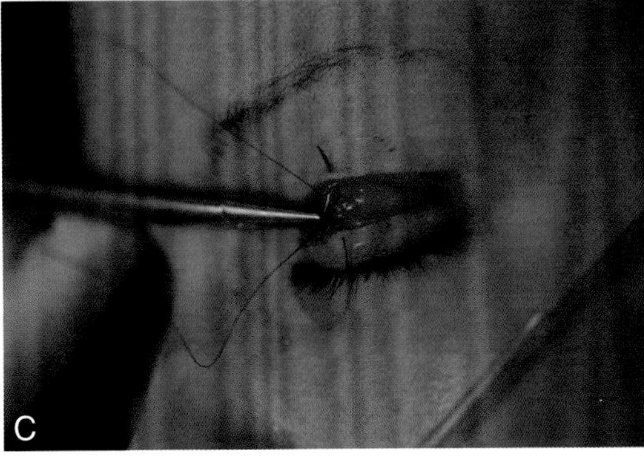

Figure 6-12. The first fixation suture using 5-0 nylon is passed through (A) the inferior skin edge, (B) horizontally through the levator aponeurosis, then (C) through the superior skin edge at the patient's midpupil.

does drip onto the levator complex, a 4 × 4 gauze should be used immediately to dab away any remaining excess.

At this point, the patient should be awakened from sedation for appropriate cooperation during placement of the fixation sutures. The first fixation suture is passed at the midpupil from lower skin edge passing inferior to superior, horizontally through the levator, and through the upper skin edge passing inferior to superior (**Figure 6-12**). A single knot of fixation is tied down and the patient is asked to open the eyes and gaze straight ahead. The desired endpoint is slight eyelash eversion, where the eyelashes are approximately at a perpendicular orientation to the skin (**Figure 6-13**). If the eyelashes appear less than perpendicular, the suture can be removed and the bite of levator positioned slightly higher. Conversely, if the eyelashes appear overly everted, the levator bite can be lowered somewhat until the desired eyelash orientation is attained. Similarly, the eyelid crease is remarked for appropriate height. If the crease appears too large, then the bite of levator can be lowered and vice versa. The reader is cautioned that with edema and the patient in the supine position, the crease height will appear higher than its ultimate position several weeks to months following the procedure.

Before continuing with the remaining fixation sutures on the same eyelid, the contralateral central fixation suture (at midpupil) should be undertaken in the exact same prescribed fashion. Besides eyelash eversion, symmetry of crease height with the other eyelid should be assessed with the patient's eyes in forward gaze. The next fixation suture is placed halfway between the lateral limbus and the lateral canthus in the same outlined manner as above. Again, the surgeon then alternates to the contralateral eyelid to place the same fixation suture and eyelash eversion and symmetry is assessed again before continuing. The third and final levator fixation suture is placed in the same alternating fashion at the medial limbus with confirmation of proper symmetry. If one side appears more edematous than the other, the crease will be artifactually raised. Accordingly, a small amount of additional anesthetic (of whatever kind) can be infiltrated into the pretarsal skin (below the inferior skin edge) to simulate edema in the less edematous side. This technique will facilitate improved assessment of symmetry during the procedure.

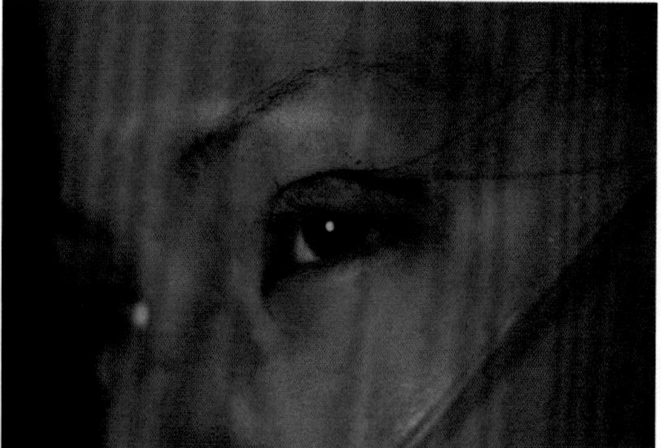

Figure 6-13. The first fixation suture is tied down with a single knot, and the patient is asked to open her eyes and gaze forward. The eyelashes should be everted to a perpendicular direction, and the levator bite repositioned as necessary until this observation is noted. The contralateral midpupillary fixation suture is undertaken in the same fashion and symmetry of the crease and eyelash position are remarked before continuing. All fixation sutures are placed in an alternating fashion.

With symmetry confirmed, the skin is closed with a running, nonlocking 7-0 nylon suture with the medial ends left untied and taped to the forehead with Steri-Strips and Mastisol to facilitate ease of removal (**Figure 6-14**). Triamcinolone acetonide 10 mg/cc 0.1–0.2 cc is infiltrated into the medial aspect of the incision line at the conclusion of the procedure to minimize the risk of hypertrophic scarring and webbing, which are more likely to occur in this region. The periorbital region is cleaned of povidone–iodine solution and blood with peroxide solution, taking care not to permit any peroxide to contact the globe. Antibiotic ointment is applied liberally to the patient's eyelids followed by an ice pack and head elevation to 30 degrees from the supine. The patient is observed for an hour prior to discharge in the care of a companion. The surgeon should evaluate the patient sitting upright prior to discharge to ensure symmetry (although at this point some edema may preclude accurate assessment) and absence of any hematoma formation.

Postoperative Care

Postoperative care is a relatively straightforward endeavor. The patient is asked to cleanse the eyelid incision with hydrogen peroxide twice daily followed by liberal application of antibiotic ointment. If the patient proves allergic to antibiotic ointment, then a suitable petroleum-based product can be substituted. During the day if the incision appears desiccated, additional ointment should be applied to maintain a moisture-rich environment. Two doses

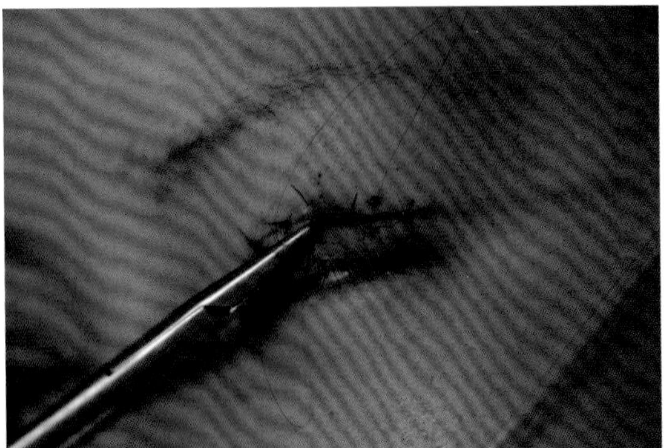

Figure 6-14. The skin is closed with a running, nonlocking 7-0 nylon suture, which is kept untied medially and secured with Steri-Strips and mastisol. Note that skin closure is undertaken only after satisfactory and symmetrical placement of all three fixation sutures, placed at the midpupil, medial limbus, and halfway between the lateral limbus and lateral canthus.

of dexamethasone 8 mg orally are given to follow the procedure one dosage 8 hours following and the second dose the following morning.

Ice packs are applied as often as possible to reduce edema. A regimen of 20 minutes on and 20 minutes off is a standard practice in the first 48–72 hours to help reduce unwanted edema and minimize related ecchymosis. The patient is also asked to sleep in a semi-inclined recumbency in order to further enhance reduction of edema if possible for the first two to three nights. Excessive exercise should be avoided especially during the first week or two to lessen edema.

With levator fixation, the individual may complain of a tethered feeling during eye opening that will dissipate generally in the first few days to a week. Also, the patient may experience pseudoptosis due to temporary levator dysfunction that could last even several weeks or due to excessive edema of the upper eyelid, or a combination of both factors. If levator dysfunction is suspected, eyelid-opening exercises can be undertaken several times a day until resolution of the condition. Using removable contact lenses is strictly forbidden the first 7–10 days to avoid disruption of the suture line that may be engendered during removal and insertion of the contact lens. Eyeglasses should be worn instead as a substitute. The patient is always counseled that the eyelids may appear more grossly edematous on the second or third postoperative day, a phenomenon observed following most surgical endeavors of the face.

The patient returns on the seventh postoperative day to remove all fixation and skin-closure sutures and is reminded to cease using any further peroxide or antibiotic ointment thereafter. Generally, I see my patients after the 1-week suture removal session approximately at 1 month, 3 months, 6 months, and 1 year following the procedure to document the ongoing resolution of edema, which really does take approximately 1 year for all the subtle signs of edema to dissipate fully (**Figure 6-15**).

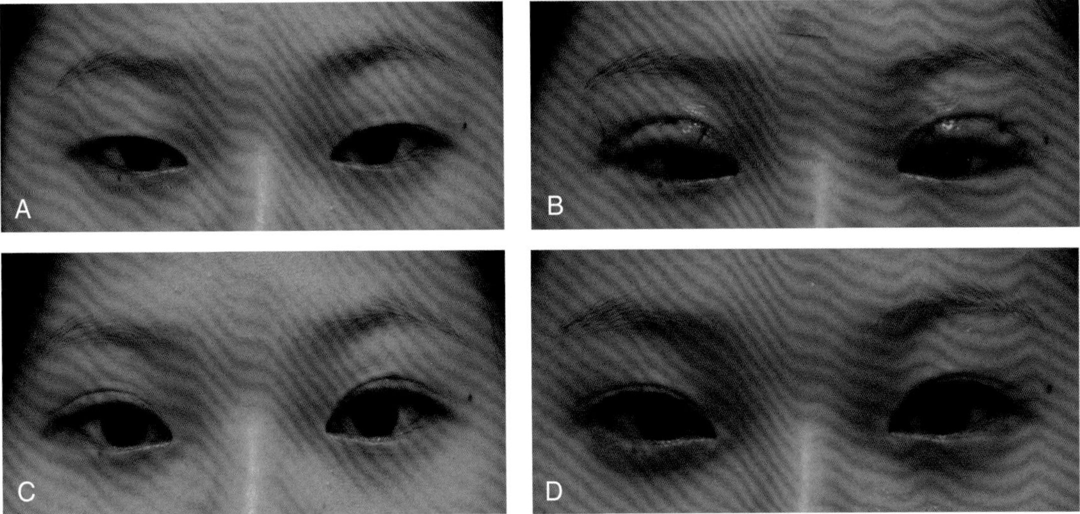

Figure 6-15. This 13-year-old Korean girl who underwent Asian blepharoplasty is shown (A) preoperatively, (B) 1 week postoperatively, (C) 2 weeks postoperatively, and (D) 1 month postoperatively with ongoing resolution of edema.

Complications

Asymmetry

The most common complication that can arise is asymmetry of the two creases. Perhaps the first order of business is to review preoperative photographs and chart notations as to whether the patient was observed to have a preexisting asymmetry. Although preoperative asymmetry at times can actually be corrected, sometimes the condition simply cannot, which hopefully was carefully explained to the patient beforehand. Reviewing these matters again with the patient afterwards is a wise approach.

If gross asymmetry is noted at the first postoperative week visit (which the patient did not have preoperatively), the patient is asked to return the following week to reassess. If marked asymmetry remains at this point, it is advisable to undertake revision surgery when the planes of dissection are still relatively easy to identify and easy to dissect apart with just blunt dissection. Undertaking early revision surgery with blunt dissection minimizes the risk of inadvertent levator injury that may arise from sharp dissection necessary after the second postoperative week.

If only mild asymmetry is present, the result could be present owing to immediate postoperative edema. If asymmetry persists following the second postoperative week, the surgeon should cautiously follow the patient monthly until resolution. Oftentimes, mild asymmetry becomes almost negligible to none over time as edema resolves. If any asymmetry persists after 6 months to a year, the surgeon can discuss with the patient one of two options. The simpler option is removal of skin above the created crease on the lower side to approximate the higher crease of the contralateral side, as it is almost impossible to lower the crease. Alternatively, a revision procedure can be undertaken by redoing both sides. It is almost impossible to ensure symmetry when working only on one eyelid during a revision procedure. It is also very difficult, as mentioned, to lower an eyelid crease that is too high. In that circumstance, it is always advisable to wait patiently for a minimum of a year, as edema does take at least a full year to resolve entirely.

Fold Loss

Fold loss is uncommon after the full-incision method but is relatively more prevalent with an abbreviated, partial-incision technique or even more so with the nonincisional suture-based method. Nevertheless, fold loss can still arise and does so more commonly along the lateral extent of the crease. Accordingly, the lateral fixation suture must be placed sufficiently laterally and tenaciously to maintain permanence. With fold loss, it is necessary to return to the operative suite to undertake bilateral revision surgery to ensure proper symmetry. If the fold loss only appears in the very lateral extent of the crease, a smaller incision can be undertaken on the one side to attempt a limited revision procedure and single fixation suture. However, this technique is not always successful.

Inappropriate Crease Height

If the crease height appears too low, the surgeon can actually easily raise the crease height by removing a conservative amount of skin above the crease without need for formal identification and fixation of the levator. The reader again is cautioned that a very low to nonobserved crease is acceptable and preferred in the male patient in almost every circumstance. Too high or sculpted a crease (even at times a low crease) can feminize a face too dramatically and unfavorably. As mentioned, if the crease height appears too high for the patient's desire, the surgeon should wait at least a year prior to revision surgery to permit all edema that can artifactually raise the eyelid crease to dissipate. If the eyelid crease appears still too high, then fat grafting at times can help lower the crease somewhat in the patient that would benefit from this treatment. Revision surgery to lower a high crease is very difficult and variable in success. The patient should be fully cognizant of this fact before embarking on this potentially elusive goal. Fortunately, for a young patient, dermatochalasis, brow ptosis, and fat involution will often continue to improve an aesthetic result that may initially be deemed too high. This outcome obviously requires quite some time and further aging before occurring, if at all.

Scarring

Scarring is relatively rare in a full-incision technique, especially when a conservative amount of skin is removed during creation of a small supratarsal crease. Nevertheless, hypertrophic scarring and webbing can still occur and most likely will arise in the medial aspect of the incision line. Prophylactic injection of 0.1–0.2 cc of triamcinolone acetonide 10 mg/cc into the medial extent of the incision line at the close of the operation can help minimize this outcome. If scarring should develop, then a combination of

5-fluorouracil and triamcinolone acetonide 10 mg/cc can be injected on a monthly basis until resolution. Revision surgery is fraught with exacerbation of the condition. Z-plasty intervention is occasionally fruitful in ameliorating the problem but still may fail to do so. Persistent erythema and hyperpigmentation is unfortunately more common in the Asian patient who is more prone to develop these manifestations but generally are self-limiting conditions, albeit still frustratingly long lasting, in duration. (Table 6-1)

Suggested Readings

1. Lam SM. Miami's double-eyelid blepharoplasty and the westernization of Japan. *Arch Facial Plastic Surge* 2002;4:201–202.
2. Fernandez LR. Double eyelid operation in the Oriental in Hawaii. *Plast Reconstr Surg* 1960;25:257–264.
3. Boo-Chai K. Plastic construction of the superior palpebral fold. *Plast Reconstr Surg* 1963;31:74–78.
4. McCurdy JA Jr., Lam SM. Cosmetic surgery of the Asian face (2nd ed.). New York: Thieme Medical Publishers, 2005.
5. McCurdy JA Jr. Upper blepharoplasty in the Asian patient: The "double eyelid" operation. *Facial Plast Surg Clin North Am* 2002;10:351–368.
6. Lam SM, Kim YK. Partial-incision technique for creation of the double eyelid. *Aesthetic Surg J.* 2003; 23:170–176.
7. Choi AK. Oriental blepharoplasty: nonincisional suture technique versus conventional incisional technique. *Facial Plast Surg.* 1994;10:67–83.

7

Periorbital Aesthetic Procedures

Paul S. Nassif, MD, FACS and Guy G. Massry, MD

Introduction

The eyes are the most striking feature on a person's face; therefore, the periorbital region is the initial area looked at by most people. With this in mind, the cosmetic surgeon must not forget to treat the periorbital skin following major ocular plastic procedures, as the skin is the primary marker for aging. Changes such as facial deflation or loss of volume and the formation of rhytides are important aspects that must be addressed when analyzing our patients. Periorbital aesthetic procedures include recreating loss of volume or facial deflation by fat grafting, by injecting fillers, and by rejuvenating the skin.

Periorbital Fat Grafting

Our understanding of the aesthetic surgical rejuvenation of the periocular region has been enhanced greatly by the advent of facial fat grafting. Previous surgical procedures have focused on lifting, tightening, and excising variable amounts of skin, muscle, and fat. This has often led to an iatrogenic skeletonization of the face and has mimicked many of the common deflational changes that occur as a consequence of normal aging. If one were to analyze the photographs of an individual in their twenties to their sixties, loss of facial volume becomes apparent. As volume is lost, soft tissue sags with its descent limited by tissue elasticity and a number of connective tissue attachments from the bony facial skeleton to the skin. These changes lead to depressions, shadows, prominences and contour irregularities that have come to define the facial aging process (**Figure 7-1**). Facial fat augmentation or grafting has developed and been refined as our understanding of these normal facial aging changes have emerged.

Much of what we understand today in regards to facial fat replacement is due to the pioneering work of Coleman and Amar. Dr. Roger Amar pioneered the concept of depositing small aliquots of fat into multiple soft tissue layers, using the facial muscular bed as a recipient site for the fat graft. This concept is referred to as fat autograft muscle injection (FAMI). The technique has increased the survival of fat and significantly reduced complications associated with the procedure.

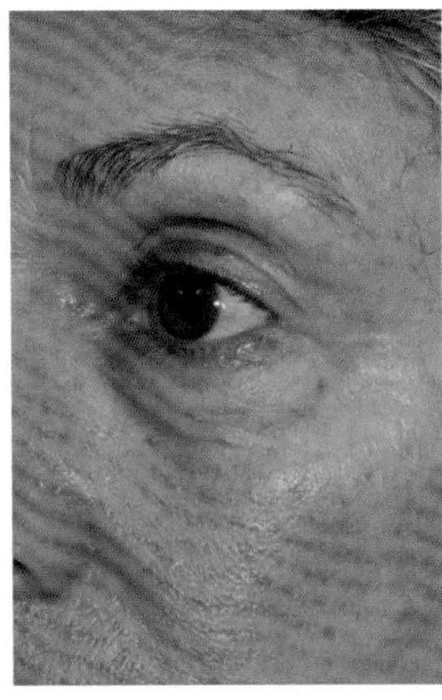

Figure 7-1. Side angle view of the typical periocular facial deflation changes leading to prominences, shadows, and contour irregularities of the lower lid/cheek continuum.

Facial Analysis & Preoperative Considerations

It is important for all aesthetic eyelid surgeons to realize that the upper and lower eyelids cannot be addressed in isolation when planning surgery. The forehead, eyebrows, upper and lower eyelids and the midface form a soft tissue continuum that must be evaluated as such in order to attain a natural and youthful appearance. The underlying bony framework must also be considered in this evaluation.

As subcutaneous soft tissue volume is lost, the brows descend and enhance fullness to the upper lids. An upper-lid blepharoplasty performed as an isolated procedure may permanently shorten the brow–lid distance and distort appearance. A brow lift and blepharoplasty (especially with overzealous tissue excision) may hollow the upper sulcus and cause the typical operated and skeletonized look. Similar changes occur in the lower eyelid and midface. As subcutaneous volume is lost, the midface drops causing thin eyelid tissue to cover the inferior orbital rim and superior face of the maxilla. This leads to a depression known as the "tear trough". When the tear trough is combined with the age-related prominence of the lower lid (pseudoherniated fat) and with descent of the midface, the typical contour irregularity, termed the double convexity of the lower eyelid midface junction occurs. The double convexity consists of the lower-lid convexity caused by pseudofat herniation, a concavity caused by the tear trough, and the convexity caused by the descended malar tissue (**Figure 7-2**).

Fat grafting corrects a portion of the aforementioned age-related periorbital changes by inflating the face and restoring volumetric proportions. If appropriate surgical procedures are selected (such as a brow lift and a blepharoplasty) in addition to fat augmentation, surgical outcomes can be enhanced.

Surgical Technique

Fat Harvesting

There are many appropriate donor sites for harvesting fat. For purposes of this discussion, the lower abdomen and inner thighs will be used as donor sites. The donor sites are marked with a surgical marker while the patient is in a standing position. These areas are emphasized secondary to their surgical simplicity. Facial fat grafting is usually performed in association with another facial surgical procedure. In instances when fat grafting is performed with other periorbital aesthetic procedures, most patients are placed under conscious sedation or general anesthesia. The patient is placed in the supine position. Perioperative antibiotics such as 1 g of cefazolin (if not penicillin allergic) and 6–10 mg of dexamethasone are given intravenously.

The donor site is anesthetized with $^1/_4$% xylocaine with 1:400:000 epinephrine (a mixture of 10 cc of 1% xylocaine with 1:100:000 epinephrine with 30cc of normal saline). If the procedure is performed under conscious sedation or local anesthesia, increase the concentration of the injectable anesthesia (for better pain control) to $^1/_2$% xylocaine with 1:200:000 epinephrine (a mixture of 20 cc of 1% xylocaine with 1:100:000 epinephrine with 20 cc of normal saline). Basic tumescent solution may also be used if the surgeon desires.

For the lower abdomen, the incision is placed within the umbilicus (**Figure 7-3**) or at the inguinal line (**Figure 7-4**) for the inner thigh. The incision is injected with a wheel of 1% xylocaine with

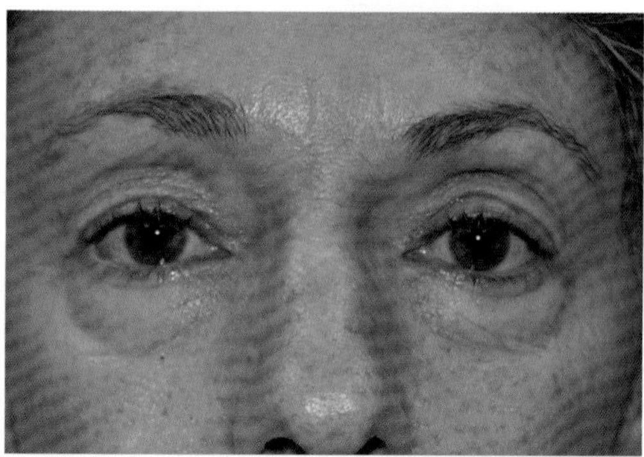

Figure 7-2. Close-up of the eyes demonstrating the development of a double convexity and tear trough as a consequence of normal facial aging.

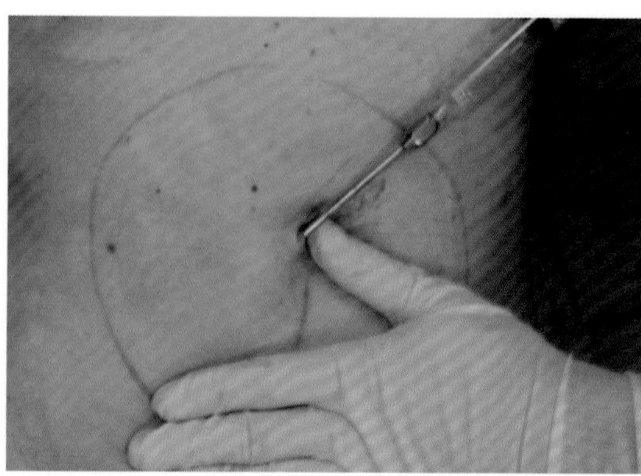

Figure 7-3. Technique of fat harvesting from the lower abdomen through an umbilical entry site.

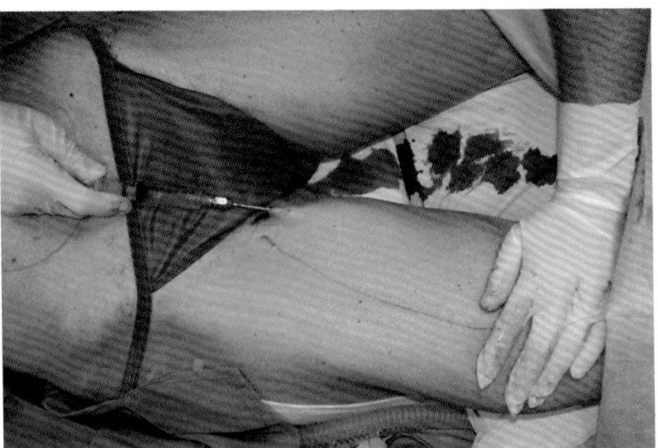

Figure 7-4. Fat harvesting from the inner thigh. The entry point should be away from the neurovascular structures.

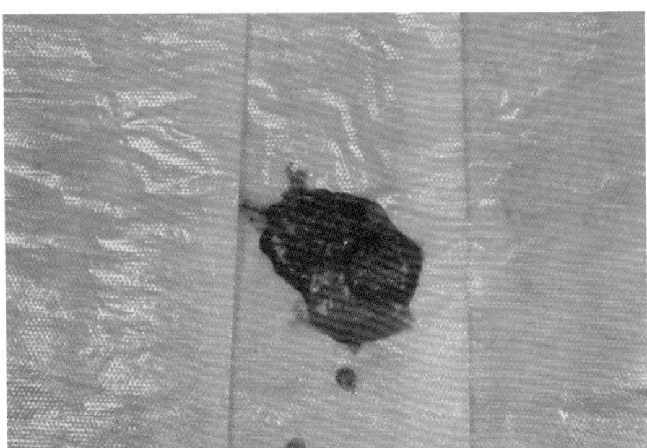

Figure 7-5. Harvested fat on Telfa pad for drainage of associated fluid.

1:100:000 epinephrine. The skin is penetrated with a scalpel blade. The appropriate diluted anesthetic is infiltrated with a 22-gauge spinal needle in a fanlike fashion in the subcutaneous tissue. The fat is harvested with a nontraumatic cannula (2 mm) Leur-Locked to a 10-cc syringe with minimal manual suction. This leads to the least trauma to fat. The fat is harvested at the midlayer of the subcutaneous tissue in a similar fanlike process as to how the anesthetic was injected. Harvesting fat in the superficial subcutaneous layer may lead to contour irregularities. In the abdomen, fat is harvested from the bilateral lower lateral quadrants. An attempt should be made to avoid harvesting fat from the lower midline, as it is more fibrous and tender (if patient is under conscious sedation or local). In the inner thigh, the skin and fascial layer is "popped" through with a scalpel. Fat is harvested in a similar fanlike process. The donor entry site is closed with 6-0 absorbable suture covered with a Steri-Strip.

The harvested fat is not processed or stored (if fat remains following grafting). Numerous publications are available to review if the cosmetic surgeon chooses to "wash" or store fat. The fat is emptied on to a Telfa pad, and all fluid is allowed to drain off the fat (**Figure 7-5**). The fat is then placed into another 10 cc syringe with the aid of a tongue depressor and directly transferred into 1 cc syringes (**Figure 7-6**). The fat is injected (grafted) with 1 cc syringes to avoid excess pressure when injecting the fat (less cell damage), and to avoid inadvertent injection of larger deposits of fat (which could decrease survival and increase contour irregularities).

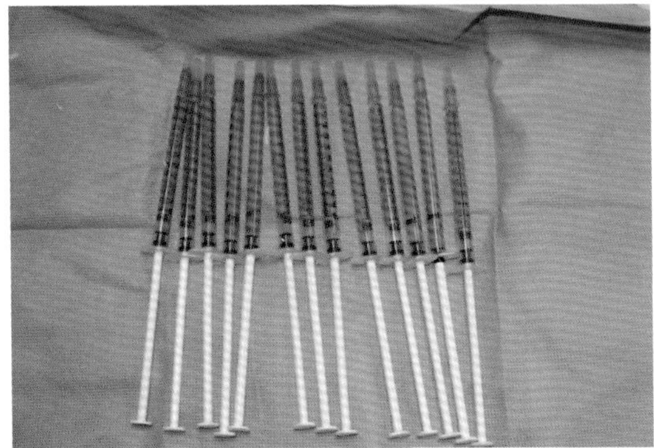

Figure 7-6. Fat preplaced into 1 cc syringes in preparation for injection.

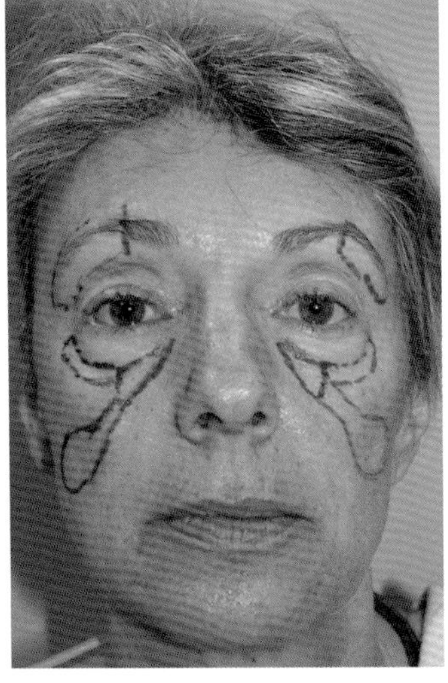

Figure 7-7. Preoperative demarcation of periocular areas to be grafted.

Fat Grafting

Prior to surgery, the areas for grafting fat are predetermined and demarcated (**Figure 7-7**).

The typical periorbital graft sites include the tear trough, inferior orbital rim, lateral canthus, and temporal two-thirds of the eyebrow (lateral to the

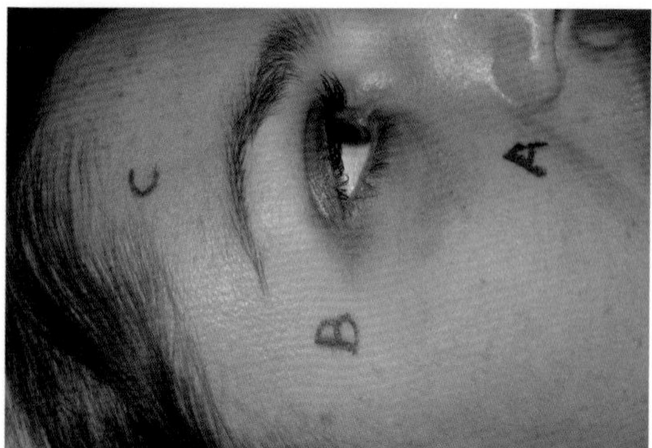

Figure 7-8. Fat injection entry sites for the periorbital area are the inferior midcheek where the alar-facial junction intersects with the midpupil (point A), approximately 2.5 cm lateral to the lateral canthus (point B), and 2.5 cm on the forehead above the lateral third of the eyebrow (point C).

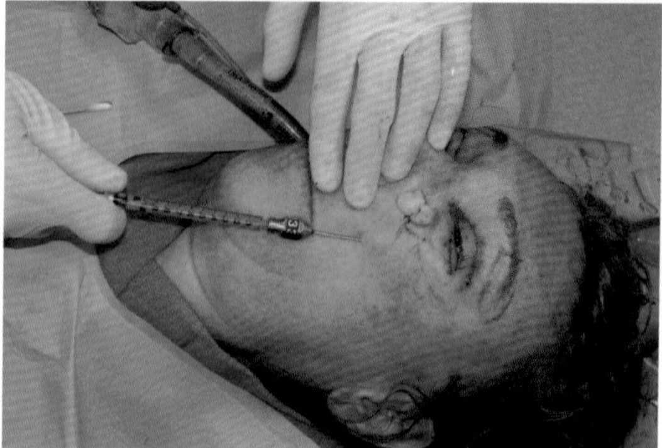

Figure 7-9. Technique of fat grafting. Fat is injected in small aliquots into multiple tissue planes to previously demarcated areas.

supraorbital neurovascular complex). For eyebrow grafting, fat is grafted above, below and at the level of the eyebrow as to avoid contour irregularities. Additionally, as the clinical condition dictates, the cheek and temporal hollow may also be augmented. Fat injection entry sites for the periorbital area are the inferior midcheek where the alar-facial junction intersect with the midpupil (point A), approximately 2.5 cm lateral to the lateral canthus (point B), and 2.5 cm on the forehead above the lateral third of the eyebrow (point C) (**Figure 7-8**). If the procedure is performed under local anesthesia, regional nerve blocks are given to the infraorbital, zygomaticotemporal, zygomaticofacial, lacrimal and supraorbital neurobundles. In addition, a wheel of anesthesia is given to the cannula entry sites. The local anesthetic is augmented as needed for pain control, paying special attention to avoiding swelling and distortion from anesthetic injection. The facial skin is entered with an 18-gauge needle. The fat is injected with multiple passes in varied tissue planes and depths (**Figure 7-9**). The deeper injections are used for volume augmentation and are more forgiving in terms of surface irregularities. When injecting in superficial planes, care must be taken to avoid contour deformities ("lumps and bumps"). We suggest advancing to superficial injections as one gains experience with the technique and outcomes. Typically 3–5 cc of fat are grafted to the tear trough and remaining inferior orbital hollow to the canthus. The lateral canthus (includes canthal angle to temporal hollow) is injected with 1–2 cc of fat. The eyebrow is injected with 2 cc of fat primarily below the brow cilia but also feathering superior to the brow and below it into the superior eyelid to attain appropriate contour. Grafting entry sites are allowed to heal by secondary intention.

Fat grafting can be performed simultaneously with a brow lift and a lower-eyelid fat repositioning. If subperiosteal fat repositioning is performed initially, fat grafting can be performed lateral to the subperiosteal dissection.

Postoperative Care

The primary postoperative issues relevant to facial fat grafting include edema, ecchymosis, flushing, and mild discomfort. The majority of edema and ecchymosis associated with periorbital fat grafting typically resolve in approximately 2–3 weeks and completely resolve in approximately 4–6 weeks. If other associated eyelid surgical procedures have been performed, this recovery time is prolonged. Often, patients feel that they have had substantial volume augmentation in the early postoperative period that is actually, in part, related to normal postoperative swelling. It is imperative to manage these observations as to avoid future dissatisfaction, as realistic expectations are imperative for an excellent clinical outcome.

The most important postoperative instructions for patients to follow include the use of frequent cold compresses for the first 72 hours after surgery, limiting physical activity, and elevating the head as much as possible for the first postoperative week. In general, postoperative discomfort is mild and can be controlled with mild analgesics. A postoperative course of oral steroids (typically a standard Solu-Medrol dose pack) is an excellent adjunct to reduce swelling. Topical ophthalmic antibiotic ointment (erythromycin) is applied to the facial and harvesting entry

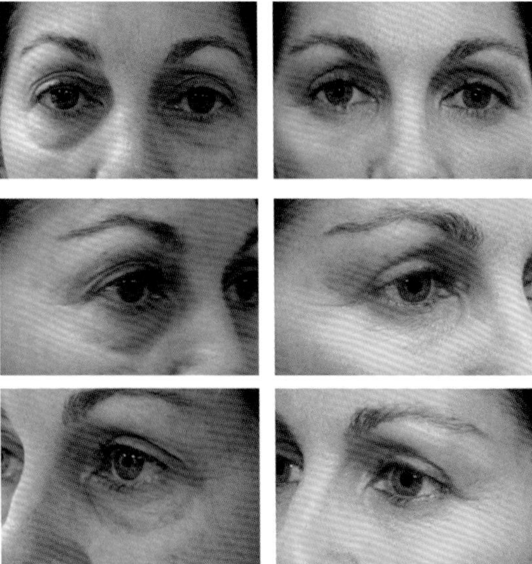

Figure 7-10. This woman presented with periorbital deflation, hollows, and prominences. She underwent four-lid blepharoplasty, subperiosteal fat repositioning to the nasal tear trough, and fat grafting to the central and temporal tear trough, lateral canthus, and brow. Note her postoperative improvement at 6 months after surgery.

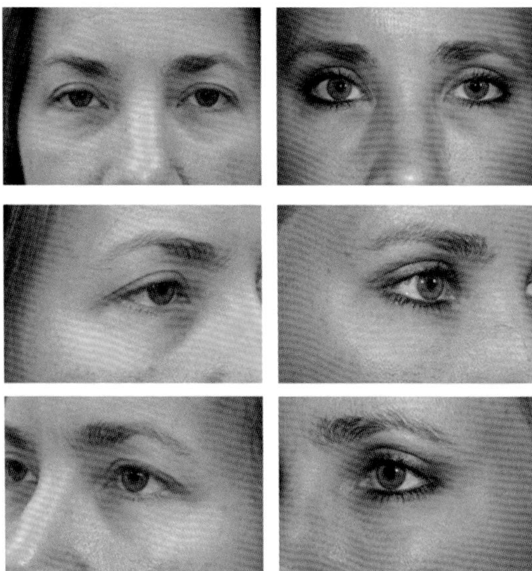

Figure 7-11. Another example of a younger woman who complained of a tired appearance. Her surgery included temporal brow lift (not to elevate but to prevent descent), upper blepharoplasty, and fat grafting to the complete tear trough, canthus, and brows. Six months after surgery she has regained a youthful and significantly improved appearance.

sites three times a day for the first three days after surgery. Postoperative oral antibiotics are not prescribed unless additional surgical procedures are performed.

Postoperative photos are taken six months following surgery **(Figures 7-10 and 7-11)**. At 6 months, the patients are informed that the current result is most likely final and if modifications or touchups are needed, they can proceed as warranted.

Complications

Complications from fat grafting primarily include prolonged edema, contour irregularities ("lumps and bumps"), overcorrection, and undercorrection. Postoperative edema may persist for months. It is important to differentiate this from overcorrection of fat grafting. Prolonged edema is usually associated with maximal swelling in the morning; a ledge at the lid/cheek junction, and on physical examination, the swelling can be compressed with creation of a depression (as fluid is displaced). This edema will resolve with time. The recovery can be hastened with reduced salt intake, continued head elevation, additional oral steroids, injectable steroids (Kenalog 5 mg/ml–0.1 cc–0.2 every 3 weeks), ultrasound, and manual compression or pressure taping as necessary. Recently, we have been using postoperative hyperbaric oxygen therapy to aid in reducing postoperative edema and ecchymosis.

Postoperative contour irregularities can be problematic. The best way to avoid them is to prevent them. Prevention is aided by injecting small amounts of fat through a small cannula (0.9 mm tip) in multiple planes. The more superficial the injections, the higher the chance of irregularities will occur. As such, avoidance of more superficial injections until experience is gained with the technique is recommended. If irregularities occur they can be initially managed with small amounts of steroid injections as described above for the treatment of edema. When the irregularities do not respond to local steroids, direct excision may be attempted. The obvious sequela to direct excision is the potential formation of a visible scar. In our limited experience, we have found that an incision placed within the tear trough typically heals well and becomes barely perceptible within 3 months.

Overcorrection of injected fat is rare. In the early postoperative period, swelling and added volume from fat grafting may worry patients as the grafted area can appear prominent. As recovery continues with edema resolution, patients are reassured and their fears subside. If, in the rare instance, there truly is an overcorrection, the area can undergo microliposuction. This can be performed under local anesthesia with a Klein 18-Gauge Capistrano liposuction cannula (HK Surgical Inc., San Clemente, CA).

Undercorrections are managed by additional staged fat grafting. This can occur as a preoperative plan when it is obvious that the patient will need a series of grafting procedures. Conversely, as it is unpredictable as to how much grafted fat will take, "touch-up" grafting may be a decision made after healing is complete as needed. The survival of fat is multifactorial and probably depends on a variety of factors, including fat quality, vascularity of recipient bed, dynamic state of the grafted area (more movement possibly less survival), systemic vascular conditions such as diabetes mellitus and hypertension, injection techniques (previously described), and a history of smoking and local pressure on the area during the healing process. In our experience, 40%–50% of grafted fat in the periocular area survives at 6 months after surgery. In most instances, patients are happy with these results, especially if preoperative realistic expectations are discussed.

Periorbital Volume Augmentation By Fillers

Fillers can also be used to restore volume and soften periorbital rhytides. In the last 5 years, there has been a dramatic increase in U.S. Food and Drug Administration (FDA)-approved filler products. Sources for the materials used may include animal, nonanimal, human, cadaveric and synthetic. The wide range of applications include treatment of fine lines, deep rhytides and folds, and more recently, facial contouring to restore volume. The use of hyaluronic acid products such as Restylane (Medicis, Scottsdale, AZ) and Juvederm (Allergan, Irvine, CA) have become increasingly popular and are used in the periorbital region. Discussion of the specifics of these products is beyond the scope of this chapter.

Periorbital volume restoration with fillers is more commonly injected into the tear trough but can also be placed into the entire periorbital region such as the lateral canthus, eyebrow, and inferior orbital rim. The injections are usually placed in the deeper layers such as the sub- or supraperiosteal level to prevent a complication or reaction.

Periorbital Skin Rejuvenation

Resurfacing

During rejuvenation, one must be careful of the eyelid skin, as it is very thin. There is no subcutaneous layer, with the epidermis being 0.04 mm thick. There are many ways to treat eyelid skin using modalities such as ablative and nonablative resurfacing or neurotoxins such as botulinum toxin. Some examples of nonablative resurfacing are intense pulsed-light rejuvenation, nonablative radio frequency rejuvenation, fractional photothermolysis, pulse dye lasers, Nd:YAG laser, and diode laser. Ablative resurfacing has been performed for many years with different types of chemical pills in addition to carbon dioxide or erbium (Er:YAG) lasers or using a combination of both. These laser modalities have been described extensively in the literature and are briefly discussed in this chapter.

Ablative resurfacing of the periorbital region offers greater clinical improvement with the consequence that the skin takes longer to heal. However, as compared to nonablative therapy, ablative therapy will give you a more immediate result. With the aging of baby boomers, growing self-awareness of our appearance, and the importance of getting back to our daily activities as soon as possible, more patients are choosing minimal downtime nonablative procedures with relatively low morbidity even though the results are usually inferior to ablative resurfacing.

Ablative Resurfacing

Ablative resurfacing procedures remove the epidermis, which is basically the destruction of the outer layers of the skin with subsequent remodeling of collagen and a regeneration of healthy epidermis through wound healing. Laser resurfacing using CO_2 or erbium lasers are target specific due to selective photothermolysis. Selective photothermolysis is a process by which selective heating is achieved using laser light absorption and heat production of the target chromophore, with heat localizing the target by pulse duration shorter than tissue's thermorelaxation time. This mechanism allows more specific targeting of tissue with generally less damage.

Periorbital ablative rejuvenation is most commonly accomplished with using the CO_2 or erbium lasers. The lower eyelid can be resurfaced safely with both laser systems with a low risk of noticeable demarcation lines.

Carbon Dioxide Laser Resurfacing

Numerous publications have shown excellent clinical results for the improvement of periorbital rhytides with a CO_2 laser (10,13–14). The CO_2 laser, which is strongly absorbed by water, emits light at 10,600 nm. In addition to tissue ablation and collagen remodeling, CO_2 lasers have the advantage of instantaneous heat-induced collagen contraction. If patients can tolerate the prolonged cutaneous erythema, CO_2 laser resurfacing usually demonstrates the best clinical improvement.

Erbium Laser Resurfacing

The erbium (Er:YAG) laser is an alternative ablative modality with a wavelength emission of 2940 nm, which has an absorption peak of water that is 16 times greater that of the CO_2 laser. The erbium laser is nearly a pure ablative laser resulting in almost no thermal damage to the dermis when energy levels are above the ablation threshold. Heat conduction to the surrounding tissue is minimal, resulting in little coagulation damage. The main advantages of the erbium laser include minimal thermal damage, faster recovery and healing, and the ability to perform precise skin removal. Disadvantages include longer operative time due to multiple passes needed to attain improvement, substantial dermal bleeding, and the lack of thermal injury-induced immediate tissue contraction. The combination of the erbium and CO_2 lasers may produce optimal clinical improvement in periorbital laser rejuvenation.

Chemical Peels

An alternative for ablative treatment is chemical peels. Resurfacing using chemical agents, such as phenol, trichloroacetic acid, and glycolic acid, as a common rejuvenating technique can achieve superficial, medium, and deep resurfacing depending on which chemical is used. The depth of penetration of the peels is agent specific and the plastic surgeon needs to be knowledgeable of these multiple caustic agents and their possible complications. A review of the different types of chemicals used to achieve different depths is beyond the scope of this article.

Complications

Proper patient selection and meticulous technique can minimize postoperative complications. Postoperative complications such as hypopigmentation, hyperpigmentation, hypertrophic scarring, cutaneous infections, and ectropion have been well described in the literature.

Nonablative Resurfacing

Nonablative resurfacing has experienced a rapid growth in the last decade. Many patients are not willing to undertake a prolonged healing period and possible complications affiliated with ablative resurfacing and therefore will settle for less optimal, often subtle results with nonablative resurfacing. Periorbital nonablative resurfacing can be performed with pulsed dye lasers, Nd:YAG lasers, diode lasers, intense pulsed light sources, nonablative radio frequency rejuvenation, and fractional photothermolysis.

Nonablative Laser Resurfacing

The pulsed dye laser with a 585-nm wavelength has been one of the most popular lasers for treating facial blood vessels and vascular malformations for many years. Histological evaluation of the periorbital skin has revealed a thickened collagen layer in the superficial dermis causing improvements in rhytides that has made the pulse dye laser a common nonablative procedure for treating periorbital rhytides.

The Nd:YAG laser is available in several wavelengths and has shown subtle improvements in rhytides after serial treatments. In a recent study, the 1450-nm diode laser provided subjective improvement in periorbital rhytides; however, it was not found to result in objective improvement.

Intense Pulsed-Light Rejuvenation

Intense pulsed-light technology has proved to be a versatile nonablative treatment modality that helps in conditions ranging from telangiectasias to rhytides. The mechanism treatment for the rhytides is nonablative photorejuvenation. Goldberg and associates showed improvement in facial rhytides following treatment with this therapy. Histologic studies have shown collagen deposition in the dermis.

Nonablative Radiofrequency Rejuvenation

Radiofrequency devices use a high-frequency electrical current to penetrate the dermis and superficial fat, causing thermal-induced collagen remodeling. Optimal benefits are achieved with multiple treatments, and results could take up to 4–6 months before they become noticeable. The most noted of the nonablative monopolar radiofrequency devices is Thermage (ThermaCool TC, Hayward, CA). The use of Thermage has recently decreased secondary to inconsistent results.

Fractional Photothermolysis

This new concept in facial rejuvenation with the benefits of using thermal injury seen in ablative rejuvenation and combining this photothermolysis with thousands of microscopic treatment zones to provide a result intermediate between the ablative and nonablative modalities. There are numerous studies are pending publication; however, this appears to be a promising new treatment for rejuvenation.

Periorbital Skin Rejuvenation Summary

Ablative resurfacing using CO_2 and Er:YAG laser systems have long been a standard for facial rejuvenation especially in the periorbital area. Laser resurfacing is more commonly performed rather than chemical peels for periorbital rejuvenation. Ablative resurfacing continues to yield superior results as compared to nonablative resurfacing.

The trend is toward minimally invasive rejuvenation techniques, which has reduced some of the ablative modalities in the cosmetic surgeon's practice. The results from ablative therapy are more superior then nonablative devices; however, the morbidity is higher with this modality.

Botulinum Toxin Type A

Botulinum toxin (Botox) (Botox Cosmetic; Allergan, Irvine, CA) is the premier nonsurgical therapy in minimally invasive facial rejuvenation and is the most common cosmetic procedure performed. The use of botulinum toxin is FDA approved for minimizing glabellar frown lines. The most common uses of Botox are to minimize rhytides in the glabella, foreheads, and lateral crow's feet. Other areas that have been used for Botox in the periorbital region have been for treatment of lower eyelid rhytides by injecting into the lateral preseptal orbicularis oculi. This injection may also cause lateral eyebrow elevation. Another use of this chemodenervation treatment has been used as an adjuvant therapy for brow and eyelid rejuvenation. The mechanisms of Botox have already been well described and are widely discussed. The mechanism of the affects with the paralytic effects of Botox is caused by the inhibition of presynaptic acetylcholine release at the neuromuscular junction. The effects are thus related with the peak effect 5–7 days after injection. The duration of action is determined to range approximately from 3-8 months approximately, with regeneration of the new motor end plates resulting in reversible paralysis. Repeated applications in the same muscle over time have been implicated to produce a disuse atrophy that can eliminate or reduce facial rhytides. In addition, there is evidence that with continued dosage of Botox, the time interval between treatment increases secondary to disuse atrophy. The most common uses of Botox as a treatment for the reduction of periorbital rhytides include the vertical glabellar frown lines and the lateral canthal rhytides. For the glabellar region, five injections are usually given across the glabella into the corrugator and procerus muscles for a total of 20 units (**Figure 7-12**). Each injection site equals 4 units (4 units/0.1 ml). For lateral rhytides or crow's feet, four injection sites are used with an average dose of 8–10 units for each side (**Figure 7-13**). These injections are placed into the lateral orbicularis oculi muscle and lateral to the

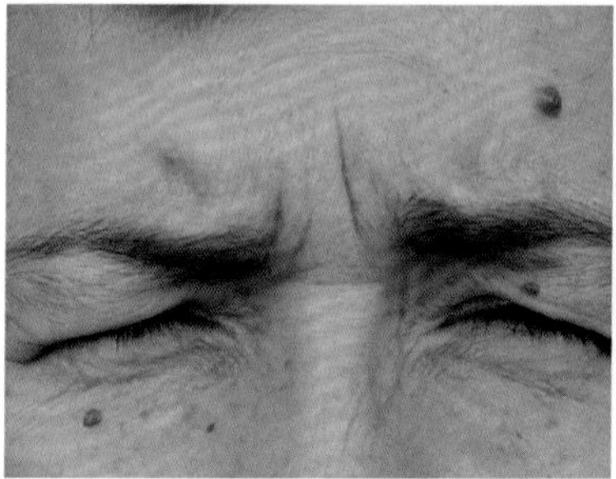

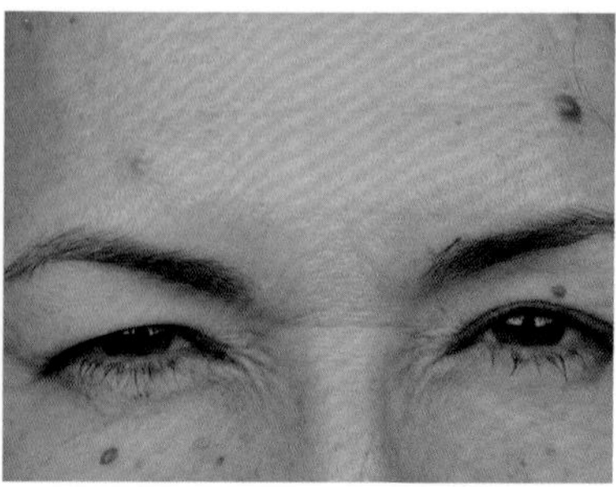

Figure 7-12. Glabellar Botox with five injections into the corrugator and procerus muscles for a total of 20 units. Each injection site (X) equals four units (4 units/0.1 ml).

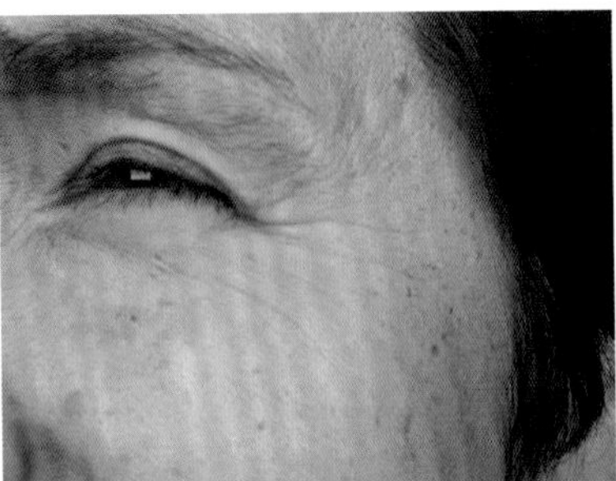
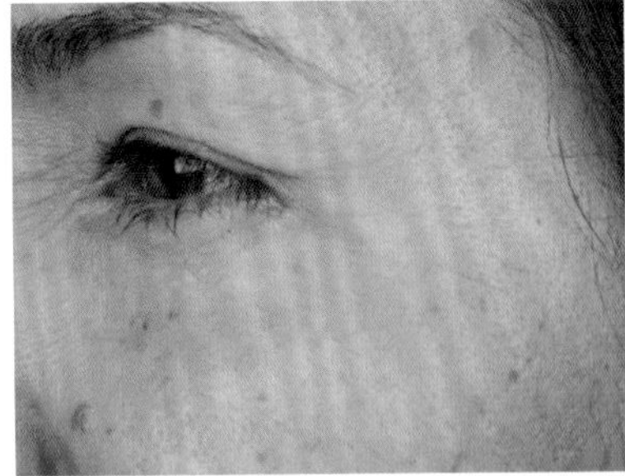

Figure 7-13. Crow's feet Botox with four injections into the lateral orbicular oculi for a total of 8 units. Each injection site (X) equals 2 units (2 units per 0.05 ml).

lateral canthus. For brow elevation, approximately four units are injected into two sites in the lateral brow into the lateral orbicularis oculi 4, which is located below the lateral eyebrow; however, it must be above the lateral superior orbital rim to prevent upper-eyelid ptosis (**Figure 7-14**). If performed properly, this procedure should elevate the lateral eyebrow. Additionally, elevation of the medial eyebrow has been demonstrated with injections in the glabellar region (corrugator and procerus muscles) described as a chemical medial brow lift.

Botox may be used synergistically with the surgical brow depressor musculature release in an endoscopic brow lift with an effort to weaken the inferior vector forces and promote maintenance of the newly elevated brow. Botox is used to block the depressor function of the corrugator, procerus, depressor supercilii, and lateral supraorbital orbicularis oculi muscles. Two weeks prior to surgery, patients are injected with Botox. The corrugator, procerus, and depressor supercilii muscles (medial brow depressors) are typically injected with a total of 20 units of Botox and the lateral supraorbital orbicularis oculi muscles (lateral brow depressor) are injected with 4 units of Botox on each side (**Figure 7-14**). No botulinum toxin is injected into the frontalis muscle, as it acts as the only brow elevator.

Conclusion

Periorbital deflation or loss of volume with the formation of rhytides is a common age-related phenomenon; therefore, the plastic surgeon must not forget to treat the periorbital region. These problems can be treated with fat grafting or fillers and by rejuvenating the skin. The modalities to enhance the periorbital region are numerous and each surgeon should have these skills present in their armamentarium.

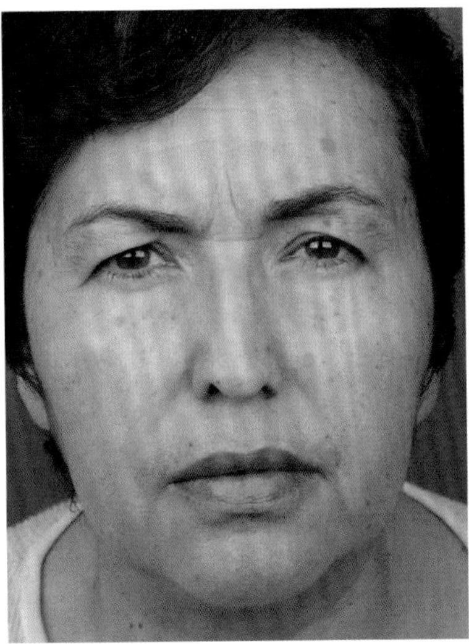
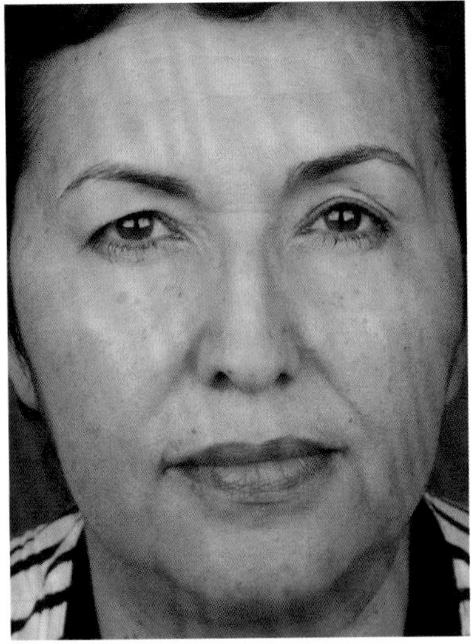

Figure 7-14. Lateral brow elevation achieved with two Botox injections into the supraorbital lateral orbicularis oculi muscle, which is located below the lateral eyebrow; however, it must be above the lateral superior orbital rim to prevent upper eyelid ptosis. Each injection site (X) equals 2 units (2 units/0.05 ml).

Suggested Readings

1. Coleman SR. Facial recontouring with lipostructure in clinics in plastic surgery.1. *Facial Aesthet Surg* 1997; 24:347–368
2. Schiller JD, Bosnial S. Blepharoplasty: Conventional and incisional laser techniques. In: Mauriello, JA, ed. Unfavorable Results of Eyelid and Lacrimal Surgery. Boston: Butterworth-Heinemann, 2000. pp. 3–10.
3. Hamra ST. Frequent facelift sequelae: Hollow eyes and the lateral sweep: Cause and repair. *Plast Reconstr Surg* 1998;102:1658–1666.
4. Baylis HI, Long JA, Groth MJ. Transconjunctival lower eyelid blepharoplasty. Techniques and complications. *Ophthalmology* 1989;96:1027–1032.
5. Lam SM, Glasgold MJ, Glasgold RA. Complimentary fat grafting. Chapter 1: Aesthetics and Aging: A New Paradigm. Philadelphia: Lippincott Williams and Wilkins, 2007, pp. 1–11.
6. Coleman SR. Structural lipoaugmentation. In: Narins RS, ed. Safe Liposuction and Fat Transfer. New York: Marcel Dekker, 2003, pp. 409–423.
7. Kikkawa DO, Lemke BN, Dortzbach RK. Relations of the superficial musculoaponeurotic system to the orbit and characterization of the orbitomalar ligament. *Ophthalmic Plast Reconstr Surg* 1996;12:77–88.
8. Nassif PS. Lower blepharoplasty: transconjunctival fat repositioning. *Facial Plast Surg Clin N Am* 2005; 13:553–559.
9. Manaloto RMP, Alster TS, Periorbital Rejuvenation: a review of dermatologic treatments. *Dermatol Surg* 1999;25:1–9.
10. Fitzpatrick R, Goldman M, Satur N, et al. Pulsed carbon dioxide laser resurfacing of photoaged skin. *Arch Dermatol* 1996;132:395–402.
11. Anderson RR, Parris RR, Selective photothermolysis: precise microsurgery by selective absorption of pulsed radiation. *Science* 1983;220:524–527.
12. Airan LE. Hruza G. Current lasers in skin resurfacing. *Facial Plast Surg Cling North Am* 2005;13:127–139.
13. Alster T. Comparison of two high-energy pulsed carbon dioxide lasers in the treatment of periorbital rhytides. *Dermatol Surg* 1996;22:541–545.
14. Waldroff HA, Kauvar ANB, RG. Skin resurfacing of fine to deep rhytides using char-free carbon dioxide laser in 47 patients. *Dermatol Surg* 1995;11:940–946.
15. Fitzpatrick RE, Rostan EF, Marchell N. Collagen tightening induced by carbon dioxide laser versus erbium:YAG laser. *Laser Surg Med* 2000;27:395–403.
16. Hale GM, Querry MR, Optical constants of water in the 200-nm to 200-um wavelength region. *Appl Opt* 1973;12:555–563.
17. Walsh JT, Flotte TJ , Deutsch TF. Er:YAG laser ablation of tissue: Effect of pulsed duration and tissue type on thermal damage. *Lasers Surg Med* 1989;9:314–326.
18. Kaufmann R, Hartmann A, Hibst R, Cutting and skin-ablative properties of pulsed mid-infrared laser surgery. *J Dermatol Surg Oncol* 1994;20:112–118.
19. Kaufmann R, Hibst R. Pulsed 2.94-um erbium: YAG laser skin ablation: experimental results and first clinical application. *Clin Exp Dermatol* 1990;15:389–393.
20. Kaufmann R, Hibst R. Pulsed Er:YAG and 308 nm UV excimer laser: An in vitro and in vivo study of skin—Ablative effects. *Laser Surg Med* 1989;9:132–140.
21. Goldberg DJ. How effective is the Er:YAG laser? *Skin Aging* 2001;9:18–26.
22. Bernstein LJ , Kauvar ANB, Grossman MC, et al. The short- and long-term side effects of carbon dioxide laser resurfacing. *Dermatol Surg* 1997;23: 519–525.
23. Sriprachya-Anunt S, Fitzpatrick RE, Goldman MP, et al. Infections complicating pulsed carbon dioxide laser resurfacing for photoaged facial skin. *Dermatol Surg* 1997;23:527.
24. Nanni CA, Alster TS. Complications of carbon dioxide laser resurfacing: An evaluation of 500 patients. *Dermatol Surg* 1998;24:315.
25. Zelickson BD, Kilme SL, Bernstein E, et al. Pulsed dye laser therapy for sun damaged skin. Laser Surg Med 1999;25:229–236.
26. Dayan SH, Vartanian AJ, Menaker G, et al. Nonablative laser resurfacing using the long pulse(1064 mm) Nd:YAG laser. *Arch Facial Plast Surg* 2003;5: 310–315.
27. Kopera D, Smolle J, Kaddu S, et al. Nonablative laser treatment of wrinkles: Meeting the objective? Assessment by 25 dermatologists. *Br J Dermatol* 2004; 150:936–939.
28. Goldberg DJ, Cutler KB. Nonablative treatment of rhytids with intense pulsed light. *Laser Surg Med* 2000;26:196–200.
29. Negishi K, Wakamatsu S, Kushikata N, et al. Full face photorejuvenation of photodamaged skin by intense pulsed light with integrated contact cooling: Initial experiences in Asian patients. *Laser Surg Med* 2002;30:298--305.
30. Carruthers J, Fagien S, Matarasso SL. Consenus recommendations on the use of botulinum toxin type A in facial aesthetics. *Plast Reconstr Surg* 2004;114 (6Suppl):1S–22S.
31. Zimbler MS, Nassif PS. Adjunctive applications of botulinum toxin in facial aesthetics surgery. *Plastic Surg Clin N Am* 2003;11(4):477–482.
32. Fagien S. Botox for the treatment of dynamic and hyperkinetic facial lines and furrows: adjunctive use in facial aesthetic surgery. *Plast Reconstr Surg* 1999; 103(2):701–713.
33. Chen AH, Frankel AS. Altering brow contour with botulinum toxin. *Facial Plast Surg Clin North Am* 2003;11(4):457–64.
34. Fagein S, Brandt FS. Primary and adjunctive use of botulinum type A (Botox) in facial surgery. *Clin Plast Surg* 2001;28:127.
35. Frankel AS, Kamer FM. Chemical browlift. *Arch Otolaryngol Head Neck Surg* 1998;124:321–323.

8

Diagnosis and Management of Ptosis in the Blepharoplasty Patient

Marc J. Hirschbein, MD, FACS

Ptosis is the drooping or sagging of a body part, from the Greek "to fall." Eyelid ptosis is defined as an abnormally low margin of the upper eyelid. This may or may not be associated with dermatochalasis, or excess eyelid skin. These changes can interfere with reading, driving, athletics, and other activities of daily living. Ptosis gives the face an aging look and can cause chronic headaches due to frontalis muscle strain. In evaluating a patient for upper-eyelid blepharoplasty, it is imperative to identify and address any concomitant ptosis if one desires the best surgical outcomes and patient satisfaction.

Eyelid ptosis can be classified as congenital or acquired. It is also categorized as being caused by one or more of the following mechanisms: neurogenic, myogenic, aponeurotic, and mechanical. In simple terms, ptosis may be graded as mild, moderate, or severe. Severity is determined by evaluating both the margin–reflex distance (MRD-1) and the levator function (described as follows).

There are several surgical options for managing ptosis. The particular technique is largely determined by the severity of ptosis and amount of levator function.

Anatomy

The eyelid skin is the thinnest in the body with loose connective tissue devoid of fat. The main protractor of the eye is the orbicularis muscle. It is divided into orbital, preseptal, and pretarsal portions. The main upper-lid retractors are Müller's muscle and levator palpebrae superioris. The levator originates from the annulus of Zinn at the orbital apex. It travels anteriorly for 40 mm. At 10–12 mm above the superior border of the tarsus, the muscle becomes aponeurotic and inserts widely onto the anterior surface of the tarsus with fibers that extend to pretarsal orbicularis and skin. Fifteen to 20 mm above the superior tarsal border is the horizontally oriented superior transverse ligament of Whitnall. This structure redirects the levator to act in a superior-inferior direction.[3]

Directly beneath and firmly attached to the levator is Müller's muscle. It originates from the undersurface of the levator at a level equivalent to Whitnall's ligament and inserts onto the superior border of the tarsus. It is sympathetically innervated and accounts for approximately 2 mm of lid elevation. Posterior to Müller's muscle is the conjunctiva. **(Figure 8-1)**

The orbital septum separates the eyelid from the orbit. The septum originates at the arcus marginalis of the frontal bone at the superior orbital rim. It fuses with the levator aponeurosis a few millimeters above the superior tarsal border. This combined fascia forms an envelope that contains the preaponeurotic

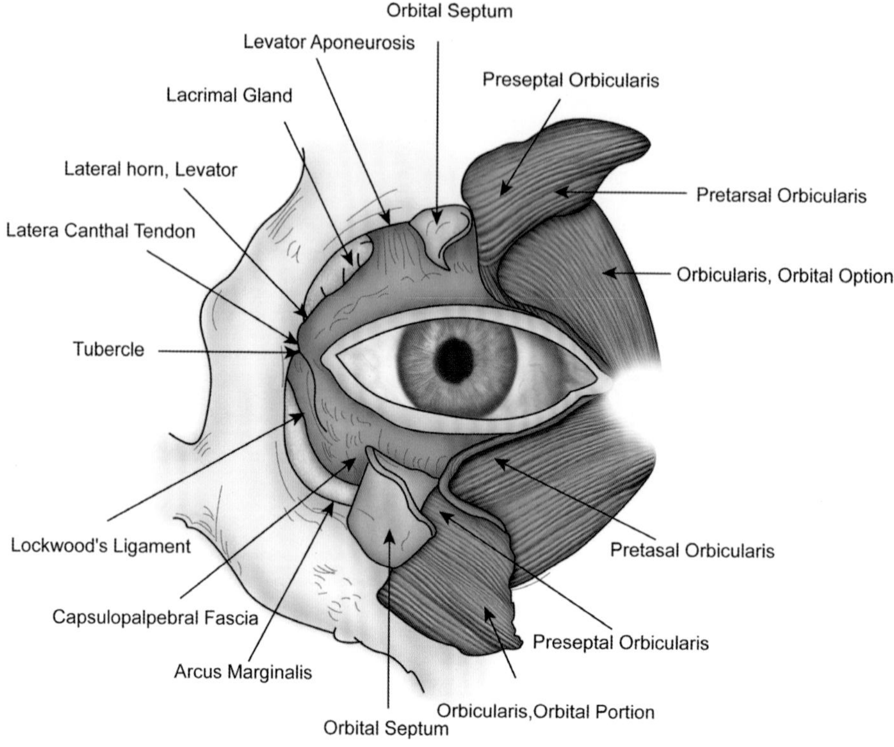

Figure 8-1. Anatomy of the eyelid.

fat. A lower fascial envelope results in a fuller lid, as seen in Asian eyelids. The septum must be opened to reach the two upper lid fat pockets. The levator is located beneath these fat pockets. Thus, intraoperative identification of the preaponeurotic fat is often the best landmark for identifying the levator aponeurosis (which itself may take on a deceiving appearance of fatty tissue in some patients).

The upper-eyelid crease is a critical structure in an aesthetically pleasing lid as well as in a successful ptosis or blepharoplasty procedure. The crease is formed from levator fibers that extend anteriorly, through orbicularis muscle, and insert into the dermis of the eyelid skin. It is 2 mm above this interdigitation where the orbital septum fuses with the aponeurosis, forming the previously mentioned fascial envelope. This fat envelope is usually 2 mm above the crease; however, crease height varies with each individual. Through proper surgical technique, it is possible to enhance the lid crease following blepharoplasty or ptosis surgery as well as to reconstruct a crease in congenital ptosis or following trauma.[4]

Measurements

The lid crease is 10–12 mm above the upper-lid margin in adult women and 7–8 mm in men. The typical vertical palpebral fissure width is 9–11 mm. The upper lid usually lays 1.0–1.5 mm below the superior limbus. The marginal reflex distance (MRD-1) is the distance from the central pupillary light reflex to the upper lid margin. Normal MRD-1 is 3.5 to 5.0 mm. Each millimeter less than 3.5 indicates 1 mm of ptosis. MRD-1 is the most accurate way of measuring the amount of ptosis. Ptosis of 1–2 mm is considered minimal or mild, 3–4 mm is moderate, and 4 mm or more is severe. Lid margins below the corneal light reflex will have a negative MRD-1 (**Figure 8-2**).

Normal levator function is at least 10 mm (excursion of levator from extreme downgaze to extreme upgaze). In most patients, even with age-related ptosis, it is usually 15 mm or higher. Levator function of 5–10 mm is moderate, and 0–4 mm is poor. Levator excursion is measured by placing a ruler in the pupillary axis and measuring the distance from

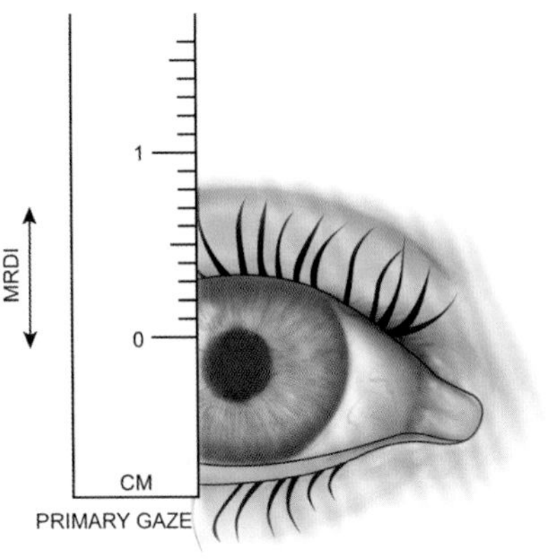

Figure 8-2. Measurement of the marginal reflex distance.

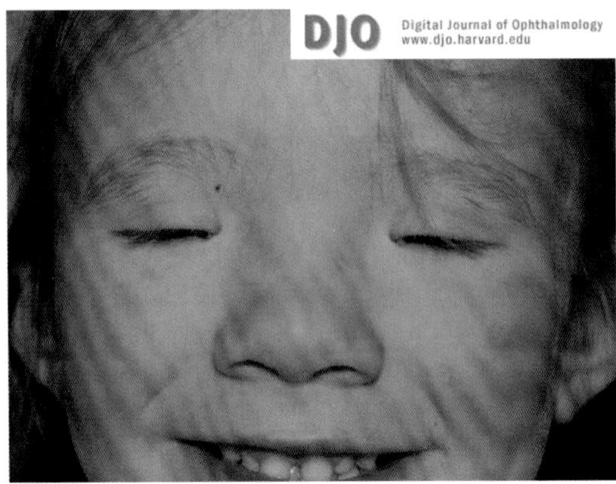

Figure 8-3. Blepharophimosis. *(Photo courtesy of Digital Journal of Ophthalmology, reprinted with permission.)*

full downgaze to upgaze. The examiners thumb is often placed on the patient's brow to prevent frontalis use.[5]

Ptosis Classification

Congenital Ptosis

Congenital ptosis results from a weakened levator muscle that cannot pull the eyelid up into position. It is characterized by a congenital maldevelopment of the levator muscle in which fibrous and fatty tissue is substituted for contractile muscle. This results in poor muscle contraction and relaxation.[2] Clinically, poor levator function with lagophthalmos on downgaze is present. Congenital ptosis is more often unilateral and sporadically inherited. It may also be associated with ipsilateral superior rectus weakness. Congenital ptosis can accompany other craniofacial syndromes or blepharophimosis syndrome. Blepharophimosis is a dominantly inherited syndrome with bilateral ptosis, epicanthus inversus, telecanthus, and lower lid ectropion (**Figure 8-3**).

Myogenic Ptosis

Myogenic ptosis can be congenital or acquired. Acquired myogenic ptosis includes myasthenia gravis, chronic progressive external ophthalmoplegia (CPEO), and myotonic dystrophy. Myasthenia often presents with asymmetric ptosis and or diplopia that worsens with fatigue. Cogan's lid twitch may be present on upgaze. CPEO may present in adolescence or early adulthood and can be familial in 50% of cases. Patients often have symmetric ptosis, decreased levator function, and ophthalmoplegia without diplopia. CPEO may be associated with retinal pigmentary abnormalities, endocrine disorders, and cardiac conduction abnormalities.[1] Corticosteroids, pregnancy, Grave's disease, and amyloidosis have also been reported to cause myogenic ptosis.[6]

Trauma is another cause of ptosis. Lid lacerations and orbital roof fractures can damage the levator muscle and decrease its ability to contract. Blunt trauma may damage the levator muscle or weaken the input from cranial nerve III. Patients may also present with iatrogenic ptosis following surgery. Sources include unplanned levator dehiscence, levator damage from cautery, improper suturing, and disruption of normal anatomy.

Neurogenic Ptosis

Most forms of neurogenic ptosis affect the third cranial nerve along its course from its nucleus to the levator complex in the orbit. They may be congenital or acquired. Third-nerve palsies can be caused by tumors, vascular lesions, inflammatory conditions, or neurotoxic disorders. Patients with these conditions present with varying degrees of ptosis and extraocular motility defects that spare the lateral rectus and superior oblique muscles (the eye will usually be down and out). Pupillary dilation may be seen with posterior communicating artery aneurysms. Third-nerve palsies with pupillary involvement or in patients who are under 50 years old deserve prompt imaging including MRI/MRA with possible cerebral angiography. A lab workup and lumbar puncture may be considered to rule out inflammatory etiologies.[1] Third-nerve palsies without pupillary involvement, when seen in a patient with known diabetes or hypertension, are more likely vasculopathic in nature.

Horner's syndrome is another cause of neurogenic ptosis. Damage along the sympathetic chain affects Müller's muscle, resulting in minimal ptosis (2–2.5 mm). There may also be subtle "reverse ptosis" with the lower lid slightly HIGHER on the affected side. Tumors, aneurysms, injuries, and inflammatory lesions are the most common causes. It is associated with miosis, anhidrosis, and, in congenital forms, iris heterochromia. In Horner's syndrome, the levator function is normal.

Ophthalmoplegic migraine, aberrant regeneration, multiple sclerosis, and traumatic ophthalmoplegia are also sources of neurogenic ptosis. Most cases of neurogenic ptosis are not treated surgically until the underlying condition is identified and stable for 9–12 months. The selected procedure is usually based on the amount of levator function.

Mechanical Ptosis

Mechanical ptosis occurs when the eyelid is too heavy for the retractor muscles to lift.[7] Eyelid tumors, most commonly lymphoma, hemangiomas, and neurofibromas, can cause ptosis. Cicatricial changes from surgery, trauma, or inflammatory disorders (trachoma, Stevens–Johnson syndrome) may result in ptosis. Dermatochalasis and brow ptosis are the most common causes of mechanical ptosis. Surgical treatment is based on removing the inciting agent-tumor, scar, or excess skin.

Aponeurotic Ptosis

Aponeurotic ptosis is the most common form of ptosis seen in most practices. It is caused by a defect in the transfer of power from the levator muscle to the eyelid. This may result from trauma, congenital defects, or most frequently, aging changes.[2] Other causes include contact lens wear, allergies, recurrent eyelid edema, and familial tendency. In aponeurotic ptosis, there is local or generalized aponeurotic stretching. The pathology is described as attenuation, stretching, dehiscence, or disinsertion (or a combination). Levator function is almost always normal (or slightly decreased), whereas the ptosis may range from mild to severe. In addition, the eyelid may be thinned and the lid crease is often elevated or indistinct (**Figure 8-4**).

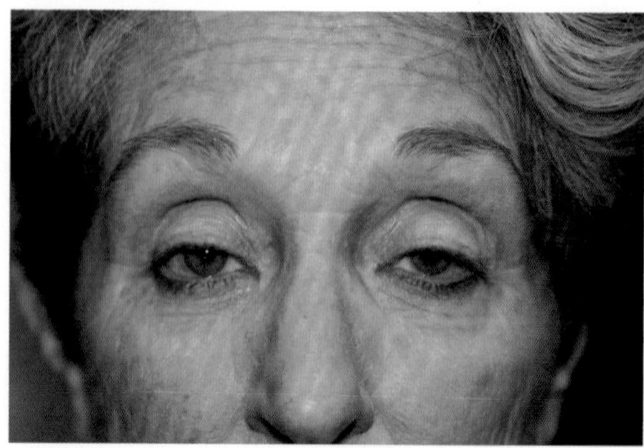

Figure 8-4. Aponeurotic ptosis.

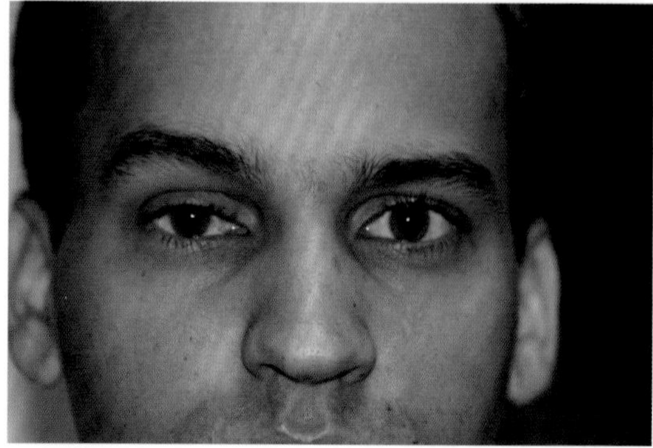

Figure 8-5. Ptosis due to 4 mm of enophthalmos on the right.

Pseudoptosis

Many conditions may masquerade as ptosis but are not actual ptosis. These diagnoses must be recognized, as surgical management may be different. Causes of pseudoptosis include contralateral lid retraction, enophthalmos, contralateral exophthalmos, hypotropia, phthisis, blepharospasm, upper-lid edema, and hemifacial spasm (**Figure 8-5**).

Patient Evaluation

History

Patients with ptosis often complain of tired or sleepy-looking eyes. They may also feel that their vision is blocked and often report holding their eyelids up with their finger to read or even to drive. If they use their forehead to help lift their lids, headaches and eyestrain are common symptoms. It is also important to inquire about family history, age of onset of ptosis, previous stroke, diabetes, trauma, surgery, diplopia, systemic weakness, variability in lid height, muscle twitches, and dysphagia. A history of dry eyes, eye irritation, tearing, and prior eye surgeries should be elicited. Patients with a history of prior LASIK surgery have a high incidence of dry eye syndrome.

Physical Exam

The clinical exam begins with simple observation. Details such as eyelid symmetry, strabismus, abnormal head posture, synkinetic movements, and proptosis are critical to determining an etiology and surgical planning. Further examination should focus on lid contour, lashes, presence and location of an eyelid crease, tear film evaluation, Schirmer's testing, the quality of Bell's phenomenon, and lagophthalmos. Especially in patients with a history of dry eyes, Schirmer testing must be documented. The test, actually a "basic secretion test" is performed as follows: the eyes are numbed with topical proparcaine or tetracaine. The fornix is dried with a cotton-tipped applicator. Tear measurement strips (various manufacturers) are positioned in the lateral third of the lower lid and left in place for 3–5 minutes. Wetting over 10 mm is normal, 5–10 mm is borderline, and less than 5 mm is dry. When possible, ophthalmic slit lamp examination can document preoperative corneal dryness. The surgical plan will be altered (see below) in patients with dry eyes.

The physical exam includes documentation of objective measurements. In addition to levator function and MRD-1, MRD-2 and palpebral fissure height are recorded. MRD-2 is the distance from the central pupillary light reflex to the lower lid margin. MRD-1 and MRD-2 should equal the palpebral fissure distance. It may occasionally be useful to measure MRD-1 in downgaze. If this is significantly decreased, the patient is likely to have a difficult time reading or walking down steps. Herring's law of reciprocal innervation to yoke muscles must be considered in cases of unilateral ptosis. The contralateral upper lid may droop intraoperatively or postoperatively once the ptotic lid is elevated. This is especially true if the operative eye is the dominant eye. This should be explained to the patient during the surgical consultation.

Some surgeons include phenylephrine testing in their preoperative evaluation. Instilling three drops of 10% phenylephrine over 5 minutes (some studies advocate 2.5% in patients with significant hypertension or cardiac disease) into the ptotic eye(s) may stimulate Müller's muscle and raise the eyelid. If ptosis improves or resolves following the drops, tightening Müller's muscle is another surgical possibility (**Figures 8-6 and 8-7**). If there is no response, levator advancement or occasionally Fasanella–Servat ptosis repair is performed.

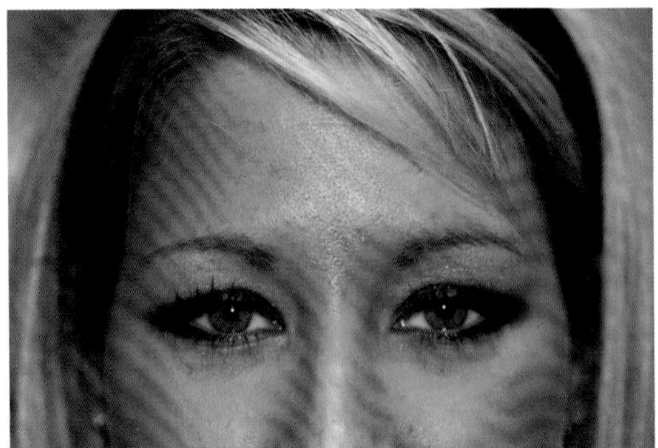

Figure 8-6. Ptosis before neo.

Visual field testing is another component of a complete ptosis evaluation. Although both components are effective, Goldmann manual kinetic visual field testing is more sensitive than Humphrey automated static testing.[1] Studies have shown that 1 mm of ptosis will correlate to 8 degrees of visual field loss.[21] The field test is performed first with both eyes at their resting position. It is sometimes repeated with both upper lids taped up. These tests reveal both the amount of field loss due to ptosis and how much visual improvement the patient may expect after surgery. Insurance companies also require field tests to document a functional reason for eyelid surgery. Visual field testing is useful in both ptosis and dermatochalasis evaluations. The required difference between the two fields varies among insurance companies and states.

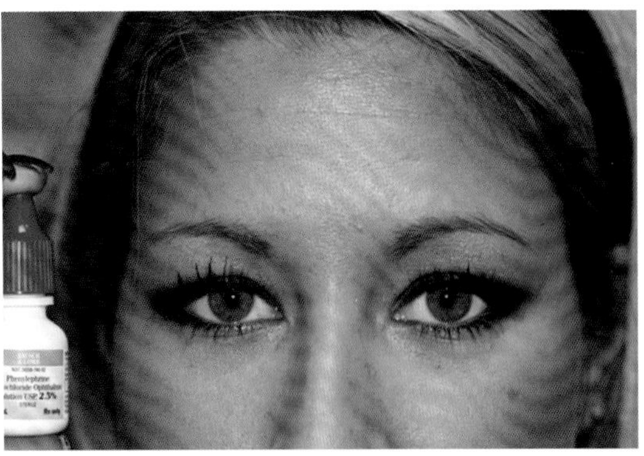

Figure 8-7. Ptosis improved after neo.

Photographic documentation is essential both preoperatively and postoperatively. Most clinicians take photos preoperatively in primary gaze, upgaze, and downgaze. If phenylephrine is used, photos are taken after instilling the drops as well. Some surgeons find it helpful to display these photos during surgery because the supine position and local anesthetic often distort subtle eyelid characteristics. It can also be helpful for the patient to bring photos of themselves when they were younger to try to recreate each patient's natural youthful look. Preop photos are also an objective way to remind dissatisfied patients of the severity of their ptosis before surgery.

Surgical Management of Ptosis in the Blepharoplasty Patient

Ptosis is almost always corrected with surgery. Although there are several different methods that may successfully treat ptosis in a given patient, it is important to avoid inappropriate surgical choices. Surgical ptosis repair can be separated into four categories: frontalis suspension, levator resection, posterior procedures, and levator aponeurosis repair or advancement. Based on the history and clinical findings, the surgeon should be able to recognize the etiology and choose the most effective and safe procedure for each patient. The choice of procedure is usually based on levator function. Poor levator function requires a frontalis suspension. Levator resection is effective for moderate function. These two conditions should not be addressed at the time of cosmetic blepharoplasty. Ptosis with good levator function may respond to aponeurotic surgery or posterior lamella procedures depending on the severity of ptosis and response to phenylephrine. These subtypes may be addressed at the time of blepharoplasty.

Ptosis Repair Procedures

Posterior Lamella Procedures

For patients with minimal ptosis (2 mm or less) and good levator function, posterior lamella procedures are effective. These include Müller's muscle-conjunctival resection and the Fasanella–Servat procedure (tarsomyectomy). If the phenylephrine test is positive in the ptotic lid or lids, a Müller's muscle conjunctival resection is the most accurate and reproducible surgical option. If the test is negative, this procedure is unpredictable, and a Fasanella–Servat should be considered. Although studies in the literature have demonstrated the safety of the conjunctival–mullerectomy procedure in patients with preexisting dry eyes, as well as with glaucoma filtering blebs, we still favor an anterior approach whenever possible in these patients.

Müller's Muscle–Conjunctival Resection

This procedure was originally described by Putterman and Urist in 1975. Müller's muscle is a primary elevator of the levator muscle. When Müller's muscle is advanced, it strengthens the posterior lamella and plicates the levator muscle. With scarring, this plication enhances the position and action of the levator, resulting in a higher eyelid position. In most cases, we prefer to utilize Müller's muscle–conjunctival resection for 2 mm or less of ptosis correction. Other surgeons use it for all amounts of ptosis because it is simple, relatively fast, and quantifiable.

Surgery is performed with the patient under local anesthesia with or without sedation. A 3-cc syringe with 2–3 ml of 2% lidocaine with 1:100,000 U of epinephrine is injected as a frontal nerve block (superior retrobulbar approach). This block should only be performed by trained personnel. A 1.25" 25 or 27 g needle is positioned transcutaneously just inside the superior orbital rim and just lateral to the supraorbital notch. The globe is gently balloted toward the inferior orbit, and the needle is advanced along the posterior orbit for approximately 1 cm. After confirming that the needle is not intravascular, local anesthetic is slowly injected. There should NOT be significant resistance to injection (difficulty injecting could mean that the sclera or globe has been entered. The needle should be withdrawn, the case discontinued, and immediate ophthalmology consultation obtained). A small amount is also injected at the central upper lid near the margin and in the lateral portion of the lid crease.

A 4-0 silk traction suture is placed centrally through partial thickness tarsus 2 mm from the lash line. The lid is everted over a Desmarres retractor. The amount of resection is determined by the phenylephrine response. If drops elevate the lid to a normal level, 8.25 mm are resected. Adding or subtracting 1 mm of resection can effect eyelid position by 0.25 to 0.50 mm. Up to 10–12 mm can be theoretically resected for 3 or more millimeters of ptosis.

A caliper is set at the predetermined amount of resection and placed at the superior border of the tarsus. Marks are placed on the conjunctiva along the lid at the level of the caliper. Alternatively, a 6-0 silk can be temporarily placed at the level of desired resection. A Putterman ptosis clamp is placed with one set of teeth on the marks and the other blade at the superior border of the tarsus. As the clamp is closed, the Desmarres retractor is simultaneously removed, leaving Müller's muscle and conjunctiva secured in the clamp. The move is somewhat analogous to the alternating foot motion of accelerator and clutch when shifting a manual transmission automobile. The amount of tissue in the clamp is visually inspected for anticipated tissue volume and symmetry, and the clamp is removed and repositioned if needed. One arm of a double armed 5-0 plain gut suture is passed 1.0 mm below the clamp with a horizontal mattress stitch in a temporal to nasal direction. The tissue in the clamp is then carefully cut with a #15 blade employing a "metal on metal" technique. Care is taken not to cut the previously placed stitches. The conjunctiva is closed using the nasal needle in a running baseball stitch in the reverse direction. Both needles are passed through the incision and pulled out the skin in the eyelid crease and tied (**Figure 8-8**). Alternatively, the needles can be internalized through the lateral edge of conjunctiva and cut short—buried within the conjunctiva. This technique carries a higher incidence of postoperative corneal abrasion. The silk suture(s) are removed, and a combination antibiotic-steroid ophthalmic ointment is placed in the eye. Postoperatively, the patient can use a combination ophthalmic drop four times a day. Artificial teardrops should be used at least four times a day as well.

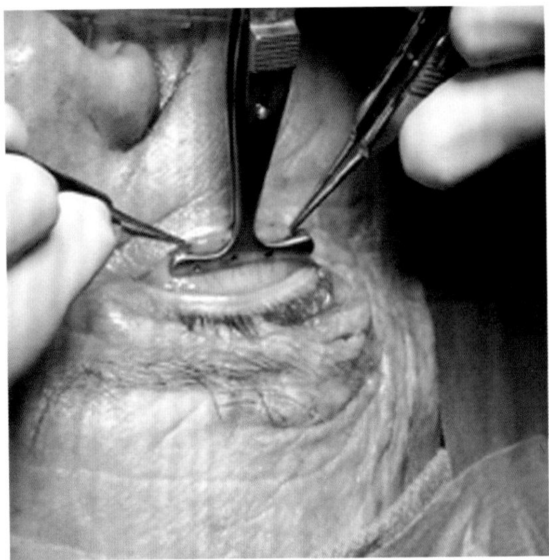

Figure 8-8. Müller's Muscle–Conjunctival Resection.

Complications

The most common complication is corneal abrasion. Other complications include entropion, lagophthalmos (rare), changes in eyelid curvature (flattening or peaking), and retrobulbar hemorrhage or globe perforation.

Fasanella–Servat

Fasanella and Servat described a tarsomyectomy procedure in 1961 for minimal ptosis with good levator function. This does not depend on phenylephrine response, as some tarsus is resected as well. We prefer to reserve this surgery for cases of mild ptosis (less than 2 mm) with an inadequate phenylephrine response. It is useful for revision of mild postoperative undercorrection. The Fasanella–Servat procedure is simple and almost as predictable as the Müller's muscle conjunctival resection. It does require removal of normal tarsus, meibomian glands, and aqueous-producing glands. Therefore, it is used with caution in patients with dry eyes and is contraindicated in patients with cicatricial conjunctival disease.[6] The procedure had fallen out of favor sometimes, as surgeons overused this procedure—resecting too much tarsus in either primary cases, or by repeat procedures in the same patient. Some surgeons also avoid this procedure due to the fact that the excised tarsus does not reform, thus decreasing the tarsal area, and removing a potential source of graft tissue if needed for future eyelid reconstruction.

The procedure was originally described using two curved hemostats placed on an everted lid, but now a modified Putterman clamp is used instead (incorporating a screw instead of a sliding-lock mechanism). Hemostats are occasionally used—particularly when an asymmetric correction (i.e., revision procedure) is incorporated. Proper hemostat positioning is required to obtain a natural lid contour (**Figure 8-9**). The procedure is begun as described above for the conjunctival muellerectomy. The Fasanella clamp is placed to include a segment of tarsus equal to the amount of ptosis to be corrected. The clamp now includes the conjunctiva, Müller's muscle, the tarsus, and levator aponeurosis. The procedure is completed as described above. Risks are similar to those described for the conjunctival muellerectomy.

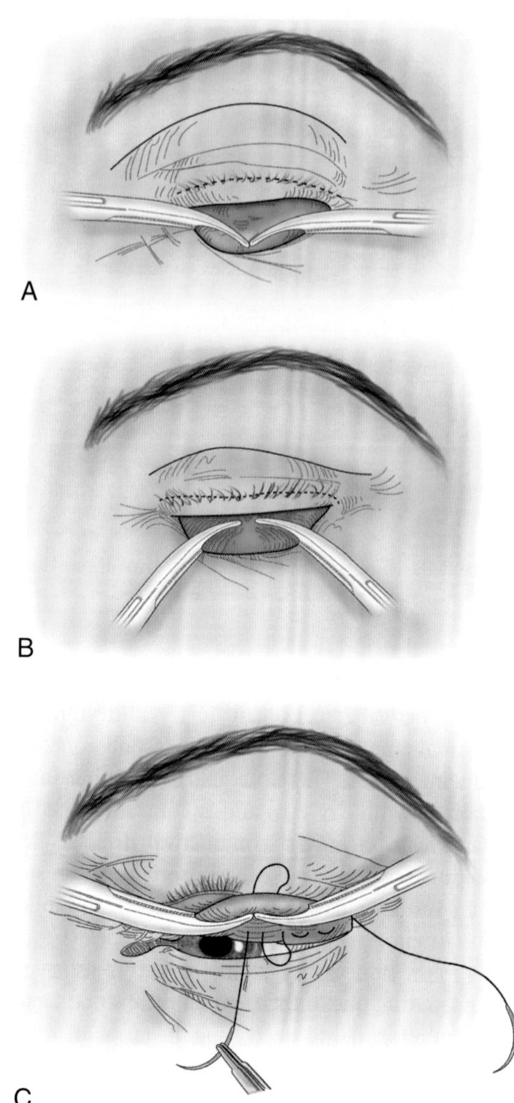

Figure 8-9. Hemostat positioning in a Fasanella.

Levator Aponeurosis Repair

Levator advancement is the most common procedure performed for all types of ptosis. As discussed earlier, the tarsal attachments of the levator aponeurosis are often stretched or dehisced in adult-acquired ptosis. The eyelid crease attachments to the orbicularis and skin usually remain intact. The goal of aponeurotic surgery is to restore the normal anatomic relationships of eyelid structures.[6] In contrast to the procedures described earlier, this surgery allows for the intraoperative evaluation of eyelid level and the adjustment of lid height and contour. This requires patient cooperation. Despite this flexibility, levator advancement is not completely predictable. Failure rates ranging from 5% to 39% have been reported.[15–17]

Many factors influence the success of levator aponeurotic surgery. Intraoperative conditions can lead to temporary elevation or depression of the lid. For example, factors that contribute to eyelid elevation include patient anxiety and epinephrine in the local anesthetic that stimulate Müller's muscle. Additionally, the local anesthetic decreases orbicularis muscle tone allowing for lid elevation. Finally, the eyelid may be higher with the patient in a supine position because the mechanical forces of brow ptosis and dermatochalasis are alleviated. On the other hand, patient discomfort and bright overhead lights cause the patient to automatically squeeze their eyes shut. Excessive sedation reduces the patient's effort in opening their eyes. Accidental anesthetic infiltration of the levator muscle leads to a lower eyelid position. Mechanical depression can also be caused by anesthetic volume, edema and hemorrhage. Finally, the contralateral eyelid may drop according to Herring's law after the ptotic lid is elevated. All of these variables may result in asymmetric or unsatisfactory eyelid position.[8] Although care is taken to minimize these inconsistencies, surgical revisions are sometimes necessary.

Variations of the levator advancement technique have evolved since Jones, Quickert, and Wobig reintroduced the external approach in 1975. Several methods are presented here.

After anesthetic drops in each eye are instilled, the natural eyelid crease is marked with a marking pen. Blepharoplasty incision lines are drawn based on the surgeon's preferred techniques. Intravenous sedation is induced prior to local anesthetic injection. Except in cases of mild ptosis (and extensive surgeon experience) levator advancement cases need to be performed under LIGHT intravenous sedation. Furthermore, anesthesia personnel should be reminded that patient cooperation will be needed 10–15 minutes into the procedure. Although we defer to anesthesia personnel for decisions regarding intravenous agents, we have had good patient cooperation by minimizing doses of intravenous fentanyl and versed and relying mainly on propofol for sedation and amnesia. After the lid is marked, 1–2 cc of 2% lidocaine with epinephrine is injected into the upper lid. An additional 0.25–0.5 cc in injected centrally above the tarsus. The entire face is then prepped and draped. In most cases, surgery is performed on both eyes in a step-by-step alternating fashion. This allows us to keep a sterile cool compress on the opposite eye to minimize swelling. A skin incision is made at the marked site with a #15 blade or cutting cautery with a fine needle tip, carbon dioxide laser, or radiofrequency device. We have found equivalent long-term results with all cutting instruments when they are used properly. Incisional CO_2 laser and radiofrequency devices show less secondary thermal tissue damage than other energy-based incisional devices. In most cases, we prefer standard surgical instrumentation with appropriate tissue handling and technique.

After incision and excision of the blepharoplasty flap (we prefer a muscle-sparing flap in most patients), dissection continues through the orbicularis until preaponeurotic fat is visualized beneath the orbital septum. The surgeon should be aware of the occasional fatty infiltration of the levator muscle (and not mistake this for preaponeurotic fat). Identification of the central fat pocket can be improved by gently pushing on the globe (causing the fat to "bulge") or by moving the lid up and down and observing for movement of the fat pocket beneath the septum. The septum can be confirmed (as opposed to the levator muscle) by its firm attachment to the arcus marginalis at the superior orbital rim (thus showing no movement when grasped and pulled inferiorly). The septum is then opened with a cautery or scissors allowing the fat to prolapse. The septum should be opened over the area of the most prominent fat prolapse. It should not be opened too close to the orbital rim—as in this location there is little room between the septum, fat, and levator muscle. If desired, fat from both the medial and lateral fat pockets can be excised and/or sculpted at this time (**Figure 8-10 to 8-13**).

The orbicularis and occasionally the levator aponeurosis are dissected off the central portion the superior tarsus. At this time, the levator is gently grasped to ensure appropriate mobility. If the levator is difficult to move, there is likely some residual septal tissue associated with the levator aponeurosis. Gentle dissection (with a Westcott-type scissor) of the remaining septum to free the aponeurosis will improve lid elevation. A 6-0 Vicryl suture on a spatula needle is passed partial thickness through the anterior superior tarsus. If the surgeon is unsure, the lid is everted to ensure that the needle has not passed full thickness through the conjunctiva. The needle is passed through the levator in a vertical manner (passing through the levator from the distal end, through the muscle itself exiting anteriorly at the desired position (usually 8–10 mm

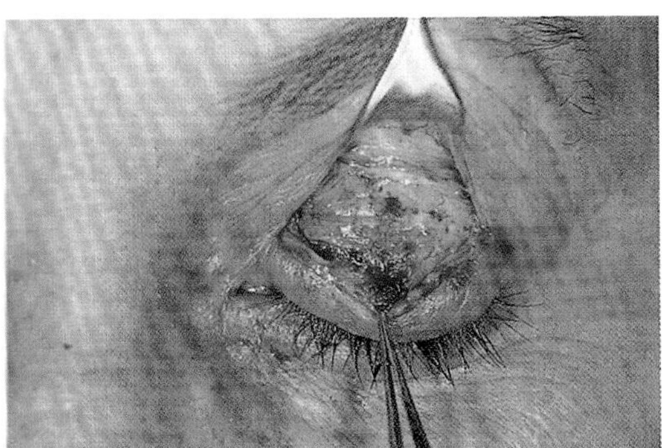

Figure 8-10. Levator aponeurosis repair.

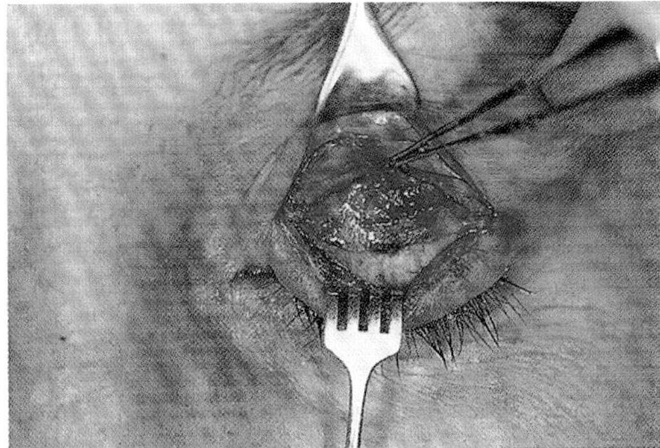

Figure 8-12. Levator aponeurosis repair.

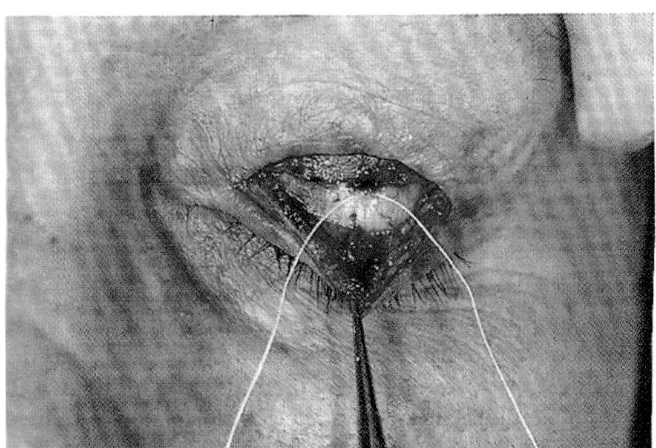

Figure 8-11. Levator aponeurosis repair.

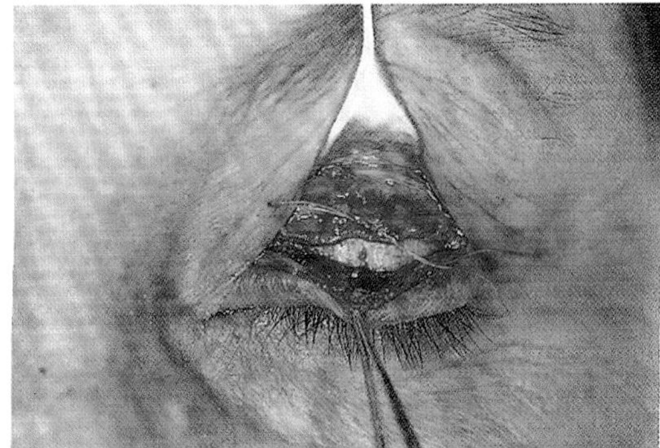

Figure 8-13. Levator aponeurosis repair.

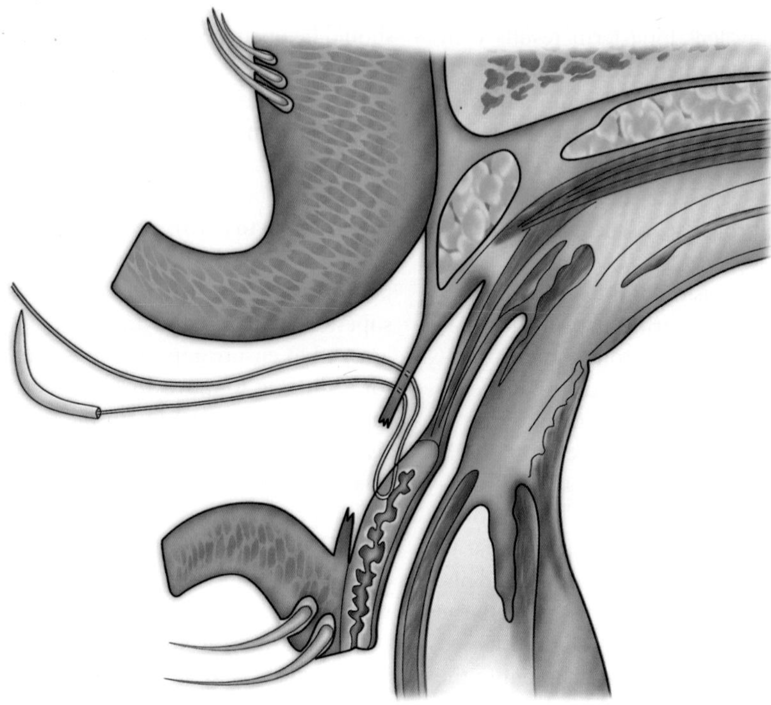

Figure 8-14. Schematic of levator aponeurosis repair.

above the edge of the levator aponeurosis) (**Figure 8-14**). This suture is tied as a temporary knot and the overhead lights are moved. Care should be taken to avoid incorporation of preaponeurotic fat into the suture closure. The patient is then asked to open and close their eyes. Some surgeons will sit the patient up at this point. If desired height and contour is achieved, the same procedure is carried out on the other lid. With both lids at the proper level, the patient opens and closes both eyes at the same time. At this time, symmetry in height and contour is evaluated. Intraoperative lagophthalmos should usually be less than 5 mm and never greater than 7 mm. The sutures on both lids are tied, and in most cases a second stitch is placed just lateral to the first in the same manner. Small tails should be left when cutting these sutures, to allow for identification if later revision is needed. If either lid is undercorrected, the suture(s) are removed and repassed, exiting at a higher point in the levator (but remaining below Whitnall's ligament). Alternatively, a horizontal mattress suture may be placed. This may give greater elevation but is more likely to result in contour abnormalities. Permanent 6-0 silk sutures may be used in severe cases, or reoperations. Overcorrection by 1 mm relative to the final desired position is recommended. After advancing the levator, the blepharoplasty is completed as described elsewhere. Antibiotic ointment or ophthalmic lubricating ointment should be placed in the operated eye(s) at the end of the procedure. The patient should be instructed to use artificial teardrops AT LEAST four times a day and use ointment in the eyes at bedtime. Due to expected visual changes, patients should be instructed not to drive for approximately 1 week after surgery.

Lid crease enhancement can be attempted by a number of techniques. Most successful is incorporating skin sutures through the orbicularis and the advanced edge of the levator (**Figure 8-15**). Alternatively, buried sutures can be placed from the underside of the pretarsal orbicularis to the cut end of the levator. Debulking the pretarsal orbicularis can accentuate the lid crease. Simple (and subtle) crease enhancement can sometimes be obtained by gently cauterizing the orbicularis just above the lower edge of the skin incision.

Complications

Undercorrection is the most common complication following levator advancement ptosis surgery. In

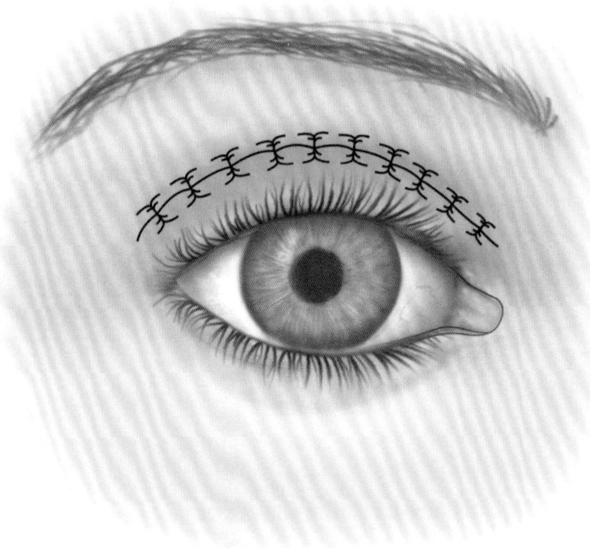

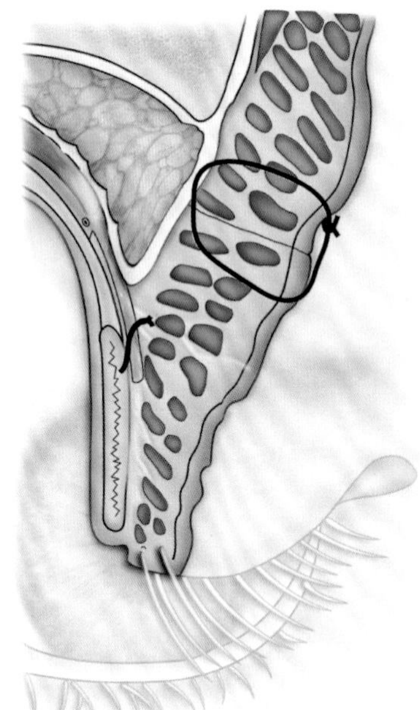

Figure 8-15. Lid crease enhancement by incorporating skin sutures through the orbicularis and the advance edge of the levator.

the early postoperative period, little intervention is helpful. If there is obvious decrease in levator function, or significant edema, a short course of oral steroids (less than 0.5 mg/kg) could be considered if there are no contraindications. Revisions should not be corrected for 3 months or longer—this allows the potential for natural improvement in lid height and improves the response of the delicate eyelid tissue to reoperation. Overcorrection is more concerning as it may be associated with lagophthalmos, exposure keratitis, corneal ulcers, and visual loss. Exposure keratopathy should be managed with aggressive lubrication, close follow-up, bandage contact lenses, punctual plugs and, in severe cases, early revision.

At the first postoperative visit (day 5–7), cases of severe overcorrection can be revised. Early revision is indicated for severe lagophthalmos, corneal exposure, or "peaking" to the lid contour. Often this can be performed with no or minimal local anesthesia. The wound can usually be partially opened with cotton-tipped applicators after suture removal. The involved levator suture(s) are identified and cut. The lid is stretched if needed. The position is inspected with the patient upright. If additional lowering of the lid height is required, a temporary silk suture can be placed through the upper lid, and taped with moderate tension to the cheek. Skin is closed prior to placement of this traction suture.

Postoperative retrobulbar hemorrhage is the least common, but most devastating complication. If sudden increase in orbital tension is noted intraoperatively, attempts should be made to identify the bleeding source. Simultaneously, an emergency lateral canthotomy and superior and/or inferior cantholysis can be performed (**Figures 8-16 and 8-17**). High-dose steroids have anecdotally shown some value in preserving vision. Urgent inpatient ophthalmology assessment and management is required at this point. To decrease all bleeding risks, patients should stop all blood thinners 2 weeks prior to surgery. If postoperative increased swelling, pain, or vision loss occurs, and is accompanied by a tense orbit, surgical wounds should be reopened and bleeding controlled. Surgical and inpatient management are again indicated.

Postoperative changes in refractive error are not uncommon. Although often temporary, rare cases may require a change in eyeglass prescription. This occurrence will likely become more concerning as the post-lasik population begins to require ptosis repair.

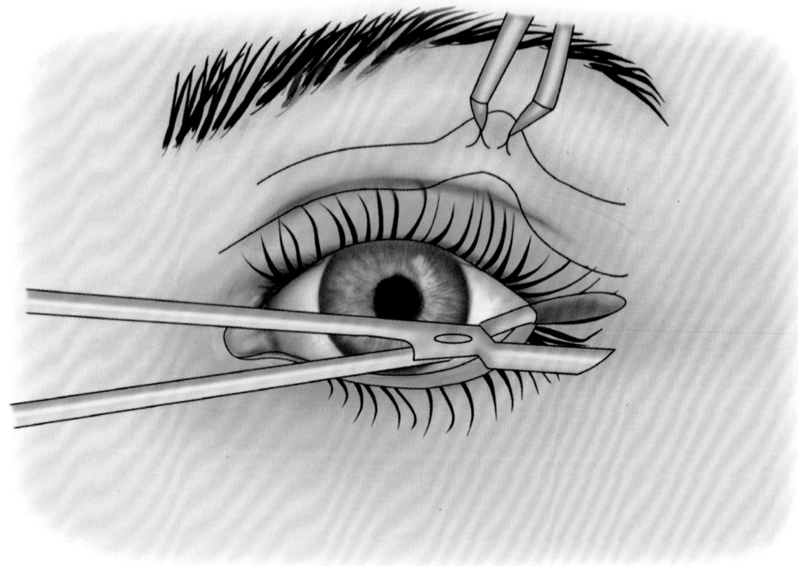

Figure 8-16. Canthotomy.

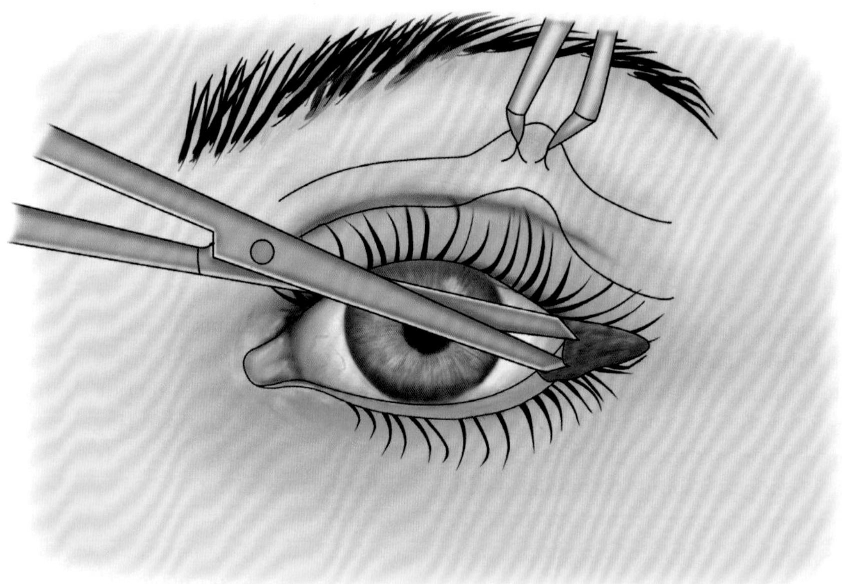

Figure 8-17. Cantholysis.

Planning and Management of Concurrent Dry Eye in the Ptosis Patient

If patients have a known history of dry eye syndrome (given in the medical history, complaints of dry eye, eye irritation, or even watery eyes, use of artificial teardrops or prescription dry eye remedies [i.e., topical cyclosporine]), decreased Schirmer's testing, and/or documented signs of corneal dryness, the following adjustments are made.

1. Mild dry eye (occasional dryness complaints, occasional teardrops (<2×/day), and minimal or absent corneal findings): Planned lid height is unchanged. Temporary, long-acting absorbable punctal plugs are placed intraoperatively. The patient is instructed to use thicker artificial tear products with greater frequency postoperatively.
2. Moderate dry eye (more frequent dryness complaints, regular teardrops (>3×/day), and/or moderate corneal findings): Planned lid height is decreased. Temporary, long-acting absorbable punctal plugs are placed intraoperatively. The patient is instructed to use thicker artificial tear products with greater frequency postoperatively.
3. Severe dry eye (severe symptoms, tear drop use >5×/day, severe corneal staining, possible use of prescription dry eye medications (i.e., topical cyclosporin): No surgery until approved by a cornea/dry eye specialist!

Conclusion

Identification and management of ptosis in the blepharoplasty patient is paramount to a successful outcome. Appropriate evaluation and surgical technique will lead to greater patient satisfaction.

Suggested Readings

1. Edmonson, BC, Wulc, AE. Ptosis evaluation and management. *Otolaryngol Clin N Am*. 2005;38:921–946.
2. Frueh, BR. The mechanistic classification of ptosis. *Ophthalmology* 1980;87:1019.
3. Doxanas, MT, Anderson, RT. *Clinical Orbital Anatomy*. Williams & Wilkins, Baltimore/London, 1984.
4. Gavaris, PT. Editor's note: The lid crease. *Adv Ophthalmic Plast Reconstr Surg* 1984;89–93.
5. Dresner, SC. Ptosis management: A practical approach. In: Chen WP, ed. *Oculoplastic Surgery: The Essentials*. Thieme, New York, 2001.
6. Putnam, JR, Nunery, WR. Blepharoptosis. In McCord, CD, Tannenbaum, M, eds. *Oculoplastic Surgery*, 3rd ed. Raven Press, Ltd., New York, 1995.
7. Finisterer, J. Ptosis: Causes, presentation, and management. *Aesthetic Plast Surg* 2003;27:193–204.
8. Dortzbach, RK, Gausas, RA, Sherman, DD. Blepharoptosis. In Dortzbach, RK, ed. *Ophthalmic Plastic Surgery: Prevention and Management of Complications*, Raven Press, Ltd., New York, 1994.
9. Older, JJ. Ptosis repair and blepharoplasty in the adult. *Ophthalmic Surg* 1995; 26:304.
10. Ahmadi, AJ, Sires, BS. Ptosis in infants and children. *Int Ophthalmol Clin* 2002;42:15–29.
11. Wong, VA, Beckingsale, PS, Oley, CA, Sullivan, TJ. Management of myogenic ptosis. *Ophthalmology*. 2002; 109:1023.
12. Dresner, SC. Further modifications of the Müller's muscle-conjunctival resection procedure for blepharoptosis. *Ophthalmic Plast Reconstr Surg* 1991; 7(2):114–122.
13. Putterman, AM, Urist, MJ. Müller's muscle-conjunctival resection. *Arch Ophthalmol* 1975;93:619–623.
14. Fasanella, RM, Servat, J. Levator resection for minimal ptosis: Another Simplified Operation. *Arch Ophthalmol* 1961;65:493–496.
15. Older, JJ. Levator aponeurosis repair for the correction of acquired ptosis: analysis of 113 procedures. *Ophthalmology* 1983;90:1056–1059.
16. Shore, JW, Bergin, DJ, Garret, SN. Results of blepharoptosis surgery with early postoperative adjustment. *Ophthalmology* 1990;97:1502.
17. Berlin, JW, Vestal, KP. Levator aponeurosis surgery. A retrospective review. *Ophthalmology* 1989;96:1033.
18. Dortzbach, RK, Kronish, JW. Early revision in the office for adults after unsatisfactory blepharoptosis correction. *Am J Ophthalmol* 1993;115:68–75.
19. Lucarelli, MJ, Lemke, BN. Small Incision External Levator Repair: Technique and Early Results. *Am J Ophthalmol* 1999;127:637–644.
20. Jordan, DR, Anderson, RL. A simple procedure for adjusting eyelid position after aponeurotic ptosis surgery. *Arch Ophthlmol* 1987;105:1288–1291.
21. Meyer, DR, Linberg, JV, Powell, SR, Odom, JV. Quantitating the superior visual field loss associated with ptosis. *Arch Ophthalmol* 1989;107:840–843.
22. Landa, M, Bedrossian, EH. Blepharoptosis. In Della Rocca RC, Bedrossian EH, Arthurs BP, eds. *Ophthalmic Plastic Surgery Decision Making and Techniques*. McGraw-Hill, New York. 2002.

9

COMPLICATIONS OF BLEPHAROPLASTY

IFEOLUMIPO O. SOFOLA, CHRISTOPHER COTE, AND IRA D. PAPEL

Blepharoplasty, when performed appropriately, is a very important tool in aesthetic facial rejuvenation. Improved aesthetics to the upper and lower eyelids adds years of youth in a region that is noted for identity and emotional expression. A plethora of procedures have evolved over the years, and indeed, new paradigms have emerged to address and rejuvenate the upper face. These involve skin excision, fat excision, fat reposition or transfer, fat injections, and use of synthetic fillers. Because complications of cosmetic blepharoplasty are thought to be relatively uncommon, their occurrence can challenge both the surgeon and the patient. A detailed and appropriate facial analysis and preoperative evaluation is essential for preventing complications of blepharoplasty. As such, an understanding of various scenarios, which predispose to complications, can help the surgeon circumvent problems and manage them if they occur. Complications of blepharoplasty can be divided into two categories: (1) general complications and (2) specific complications related to the upper and lower eyelids. In this chapter, we outline the pertinent anatomy and facial analysis and describe the related complications and their general management. For a detailed in-depth description, the reader is directed to address the appropriate texts.

Anatomy of the Eyelids

As the face of our facial plastic cosmetic practice continues to evolve to include patients of various ethnicities, and indeed various prevailing aesthetic trends, the variety and complexity of periorbital surgical procedures and potential complications also increase. The facial plastic surgeon is encouraged to have a commanding knowledge of related eyelid anatomy. In evaluating the superficial topography of the eyelids, an understanding of the ideal position of the brow is critical because this has a profound impact on the appearance of the eye below. Ideal eyebrow aesthetics has been described differently based on gender and perhaps ethnicity and culture. Typically, female eyebrows are arched with a peak whose horizontal high point is in line with the lateral limbus, approximately 1 cm above the superior orbital rim. The male eyebrow, however, is ideally less peaked and approximates the level of the superior orbital rim.

Figure 9-1 demonstrates many important anatomic relationships for the eyelids. The lateral canthus is generally 2–4 mm superior to the medial canthus. This allows the tears from the superior, laterally positioned lacrimal gland to bathe the eye and then run downhill in their medial movement to the lacrimal drainage apparatus, located in the medial canthus. The palpebral fissures in the adult average 10–12 mm vertically and 28–30 mm horizontally. The upper eyelid is positioned at or 1–2 mm below the upper limbus. The position of the upper eyelid crease varies with ethnicity. In the Caucasian upper lid, the crease is typically 7–8 mm above the margin in men and 10–12 mm above the lid margin in women. In Asians, however, the upper lid crease may be lower or altogether absent owing to a lower insertion of the septum and variable or absent insertion of the levator aponeurosis into the upper lid skin.

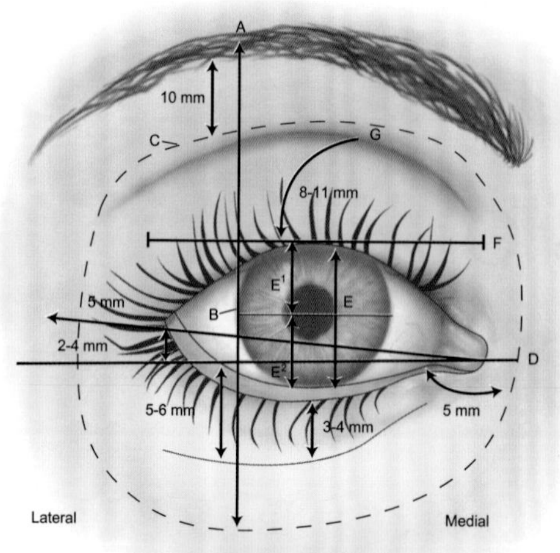

Figure 9-1. Topography of the eyelid. (A) The highest point of the brow is at or lateral to the lateral limbus. (B) The inferior edge of the brow is typically 10 mm superior to the supraorbital rim. (C) Also shown are the ranges for average palpebral height (10–12 mm), width (28–30 mm), (D) and upper lid fold (8–11 mm, with gender and racial differences). Note that the lateral canthus is ~4 mm higher than the medial canthus. (E) Intrapalpebral distance measures 10–12 mm. (E^1) Mean reflex distance (MRD) 1. (E^2) MRD 2. (F) Palpebral width. (G) Upper lid fold is 8–11 mm.

The medial and lateral canthal ligaments attach to the orbital rims medially at the anterior and posterior lacrimal crest and laterally on Whitnall's tubercle. The orbital septum is a strong sheet of connective tissue defining the anterior extent of the orbit. The septum creates a compartment through which blood cannot escape postsurgically, thus forming the "raccoon eyes" seen postoperatively. With aging, the orbital fat may prolapse through thin areas of the septum, leading to pseudoherniation of fat or steatoblepharon. The upper eyelid has two distinct fat pads separated by the superior oblique muscle: the central fat pad, which is yellow in color, and the nasal fat pad, which is firmer and paler in color. Histologically, the differences are in a greater amount of connective tissue and blood vessels in the nasal fat, whereas the central fat has a greater amount of carotenoids.

The anatomy of the lower eyelid is of particular interest because complications commonly occur in this area. As such, an understanding of normal relationships is critical to prevention and correction of these complications. The lower lid margin typically rests at or 1 mm above the inferior limbus. The lower eyelid is supported and suspended by the lateral and medial canthal tendons, the capsulopalpebral fascia, the tarsus, and the orbicularis oculi muscle. The lower eyelid is subdivided into the anterior lamella (the skin and orbicularis oculi muscle), the middle lamella (the orbital septum and orbital fat), and the posterior lamella (the capsulopalpebral fascia and conjunctiva). The orbital septum in the lower eyelid originates at the arcus marginalis along the inferior orbital rim and inserts into the capsulopalpebral fascia or lower eyelid retractors approximately 5 mm below the inferior tarsal border (**Figure 9-2**). The inferior lid has three distinct fat pads: namely, the nasal, central, and lateral fat pads. The central and nasal pads are separated by the inferior oblique muscle, a structure that must be preserved during surgery of the lower eyelid. The lower lid is continuous with the suborbicularis oculi fat (SOOF) that extends posteriorly to the orbicularis and inferiorly to the midface. Ptosis of the midface tissues thus may contribute to the appearance of the tear-trough defect. Finally, the lower eyelid is considered most aesthetically appealing when the lateral canthus is approximately 2–3 mm above a horizontal plane at the level of the medial canthus. The surgeon should always seek to maintain or restore this ideal aesthetic relationship of the lower eyelid to the globe. Careful preoperative analysis and understanding of the aesthetic ideal provides the foundation for avoiding complications of lower eyelid blepharoplasty as they relate to eyelid position and function. The reader is directed to a more detailed text for better and more complete description of the surgical anatomy of the eyelids.

Evaluation of the anatomy and marking of the patient should be done with the patient sitting in an upright position. Gravity is one of the most important culprits for the tissue changes that result in skin folding, connective tissue weakening, and fat pad prolapse. In such a position, asymmetries are noticed and compensated for, eyelid creases are noted and marked, and fat pads are outlined while identifying areas that might require fat repositioning rather than removal. Preoperative photos are critical not only for medicolegal reasons but also for a detailed study of the anatomy. A detailed study of the photos could uncover subtle anomalies such as true ptosis of the eyelids.

History and Physical Examination

As with any surgical patient, a detailed history and physical examination is of utmost importance. It is

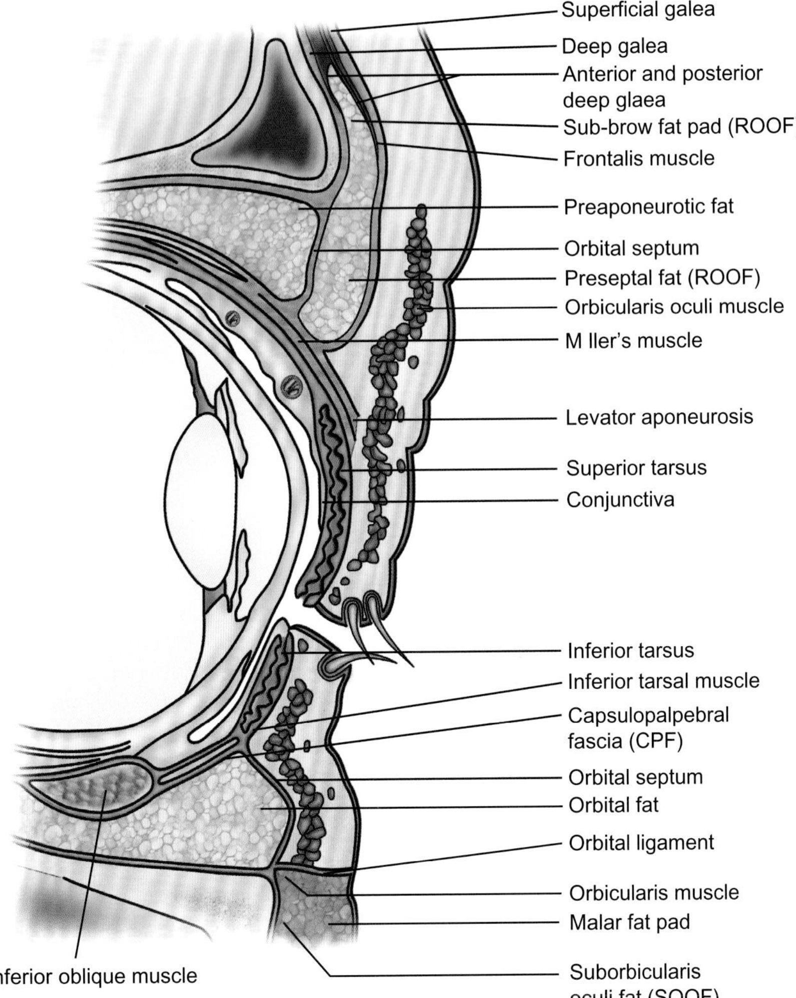

Figure 9-2. Cross-sectional anatomy of the upper and lower lids. The capsulopalpebral fascia and inferior tarsal muscle are retractors of the lower lid, whereas Müller's muscle, the levator muscle, and its aponeurosis are retractors of the upper lid. Note the preseptal positioning of the retro-orbicularis oculi (ROOF) and the suborbicularis oculi fat (SOOF). The orbitomalar ligament arises from the arcus marginalis of the inferior orbital rim and inserts on skin of the lower lid, forming the nasojugal fold.

imperative to recognize patients who could be at greater risk of complications from surgical rejuvenation of the periocular region. For this reason, it is imperative that the surgeon performs a thorough preoperative history and examination. Medical conditions such as hypertension, diabetes mellitus, smoking history, and blood dyscrasias may place the patient at higher risk for bleeding and healing issues. In addition, systemic diseases that affect the eyes may include Graves' disease and thyroid disorders, rheumatoid arthritis, systemic lupus erythromatosis, hypercholesterolemia, cardiac disease, peripheral vascular disease, atopic dermatitis, rosacea, pemphigus, Sjögren's syndrome (dry eyes), myasthenia gravis (ptosis), Bell's palsy, and other neuromuscular syndromes. Prior trauma and surgical history (including refractive surgery) as well as surgery for skin cancer are important to identify. Other important aspects of the physical examination should include a visual acuity test, visual field test, evaluation of the quality of the eyelid skin, evaluation of the cranial nerves, corneal sensation, and a Bell's phenomenon evaluation. Finally, a review of medications including herbal and alternative remedies must include identifying antiplatelet and blood thinning medications. Many of the newer psychological agents interact with the sympathomimetic amines and must be discontinued before surgery. Homeopathic medications are clearly a common part of many Americans' daily nutritional supplements. Many of these herbal preparations interact with medications used at surgery. St. John's wort, yohimbe, and licorice root can have a monoamine oxidase inhibitory effect. Gingko biloba, used for short-term memory loss, is a powerful anticoagulant. Men in this age group also commonly use medications for erectile dysfunction, which can cause severe vasodilation and a drop in blood pressure during surgery. It is best to have a patient report all medications, including alternative medications. In addition, it may help to provide a list of "do not use" medications, because some patients may not consider these remedies as medications and, as a result, may not report them.

The surgeon must also identify preoperatively patients that may have unrealistic expectations. It is estimated that up to 25% of people seeking cosmetic surgery may have body dysmorphic disorder or an unrealistic expectation of themselves. Common indicators may include dissatisfaction with prior cosmetic surgery, lofty expectations, or obsessive-compulsive tendencies. Regardless of how well surgery may go for such patients, they may continue to be unhappy with the results that may ensue. Therefore, it is worth a surgeon's investment in time with the patient preoperatively to identify such matters and either postpone or excuse himself or herself from offering a procedure to cure self-dissatisfaction. In general, preoperative identification of high-risk patients is critical to preventing complications in blepharoplasty (**Table 9-1**).

General Complications

Some complications apply to either the upper or the lower eyelid blepharoplasty. These include bleeding/hematoma, dry eyes, globe injury, corneal abrasion, changes in vision, chemosis, infection, and suture line complications. In addition, medical risks, if not identified, can contribute immensely to complications. **Table 9-2** lists possible complications of blepharoplasty.

TABLE 9-1 Preoperative Identification of High-Risk Patients

1. Dry eye syndrome/Sjögren's syndrome
2. Thyroid disease
3. Lower lid laxity
4. Negative vector
5. Scleral show
6. Previous facial trauma
7. Previous facial surgery
8. Psychological issues
9. Unrealistic expectations

TABLE 9-2 Possible Complications of Blepharoplasty

General Complications
Infection
Conjunctival chemosis
Ecchymosis
Bleeding
Retrobulbar hematoma
Wound dehiscence
Hypertropic scar
Milia
Dry eye
Corneal abrasion
Pyogenic granuloma and suture granuloma
Hyperpigmentation
Blindness

Upper Eyelid Complications
Lagophthalmos
Asymmetry of sides
Misdiagnosis of ptosis
Postoperative ptosis from levator injury
Oversculpturing with superior sulcus defect
Medial canthal webbing

Lower Eyelid Complications
Ectropion
Scleral show
Strabismus
Entropion
Lower lid retraction
Rounding of the lateral sulcus
Oversculpturing of lower lid fat with tear trough defect

Orbital Hemorrhage

Issues of bleeding may include a spectrum of possibilities such as intraoperative bleeding, subcutaneous hematomas, and orbital retrobulbar hematomas. Whereas almost every patient experiences some degree of bleeding, skin edema, and ecchymosis, a detailed preoperative evaluation and meticulous hemostasis intraoperatively helps to minimize troublesome bleeding, especially when dealing with periorbital fat. A thorough history may reveal a personal or family history of bleeding disorders, easy bruising, and other cues to an underlying disorder such as von Willebrand's disease. Further investigation of such a history and appropriate perioperative management of such disorders may significantly reduce the chances of perioperative bleeding. Most bleeding problems, however, are identified in the early postoperative period. Any patient with significant unilateral swelling of the eyelids should be carefully monitored. With a subcutaneous hematoma, the patient may not have eye pain or visual loss, and simple opening of an incision with identification of the bleeding vessel is the treatment of choice. However, if decreasing visual acuity occurs, suspect retrobulbar hematoma and immediately involve an ophthalmologist because irreversible injury can occur in as little as 90 minutes.

In addition to the possible causes of bleeding problems and hematomas listed previously, there are other commonly implicated causes that relate to the actual surgical technique. Excessive traction on orbital fat, resulting in disruption of small arterioles or venules in the posterior orbit, and failure to properly clamp and cauterize the fat and vessels with bipolar cautery prior to excision of fat is a major cause. The fat stump typically retracts into the orbit and is not easily accessed, especially in a sedated patient. Another cause is the failure to recognize an open vessel because of either vasospasm or the epinephrine effect. Direct vessel trauma resulting from injections blindly deep to the orbital septum and rebleeding after closure resulting from any maneuver or event such as a violent emergence from anesthesia that may raise ophthalmic arteriovenous pressure may result in bleeding. For this, a deliberate and direct communication with the anesthesia provider to prevent such problems is strongly advised. In the event that a violent emergence from anesthesia is encountered, the surgeon is advised to extend the postoperative observational period.

Collections of blood beneath the skin surface can usually be minimized by optimizing the patient's coagulation profiles and normotensive status during surgery. Also, delicate surgery through meticulous tissue handling, respect of tissue planes, and perhaps, use of lasers for incisions have been shown to decrease bleeding. After surgery, head elevation, cold compresses, appropriate analgesic support, and limited activity help. Should hematoma develop, its extent and time of presentation will guide management.

As mentioned previously, small and superficial hematomas are relatively common and are typically self-limiting. These typically do not require any intervention. If organization occurs with the development of an indurated mass and resolution is slow or nonprogressive, conservative steroid injections may be used to hasten the healing process. Moderate or large hematomas recognized after several days can be evacuated once recognized, or better yet allowed to liquefy, then evacuated with a large-bore needle aspiration or by creating a small stab wound over it with a no. 11 blade. Hematomas that are large and present early, are expanding, or represent symptomatic retrobulbar extension demand immediate exploration and hemostatic control. In this case, urgent ophthalmologic consultation and orbital decompression are the mainstays of management.

Blindness

Vision loss due to retrobulbar hematoma is by far the most feared complication resulting from blepharoplasty. Fortunately, the occurrence is rare, where the incidence is reportedly 0.04% or 1 in 2,500 cases. Acute retrobulbar hematoma may compress neurovascular structures, compromising retinal artery blood flow, leading to ischemia of the retina, central artery, and most importantly, the optic nerve. Symptoms in this case include severe pain, visual changes ranging from hemianopsia to amaurosis fugax, and scintillating scotomas. Examination will often reveal a tense and protuberant periorbital area with diminished or absent extraocular movements. Additional findings may include afferent papillary defect and macular changes on direct fundoscopy. Intraocular pressure must be measured because increased pressures must be identified. Pressures greater than 40 mmHg are concerning because the filling pressures of the retinal arteries are lower than this value. Once the diagnosis is made, treatment should be implemented immediately because 90–120 minutes of ischemia leads to irreversible blindness (**Figure 9-3**). Immediate intervention includes an emergent ophthalmologic consultation. In addition, opening of the suture lines to relieve pressure and possibly identify a bleeding vessel and applying iced saline compresses while the head is elevated can be effective. Further urgent medical therapy includes administration of osmotic agents, such a mannitol 20% at a dose of 1.5–2 g/kg intravenously with the first 12.5 g given over 3–5 minutes and the remainder given over a 30-minute period. Steroids such as Solu-Medrol (Pharmacia & Upjohn, New York), 100 mg intravenously, or methylprednisolone, 10 mg intravenous push, are given. Carbonic anhydrase inhibitors (acetazolamide, 500 mg, slow intravenous push) as well as topical beta-blockers

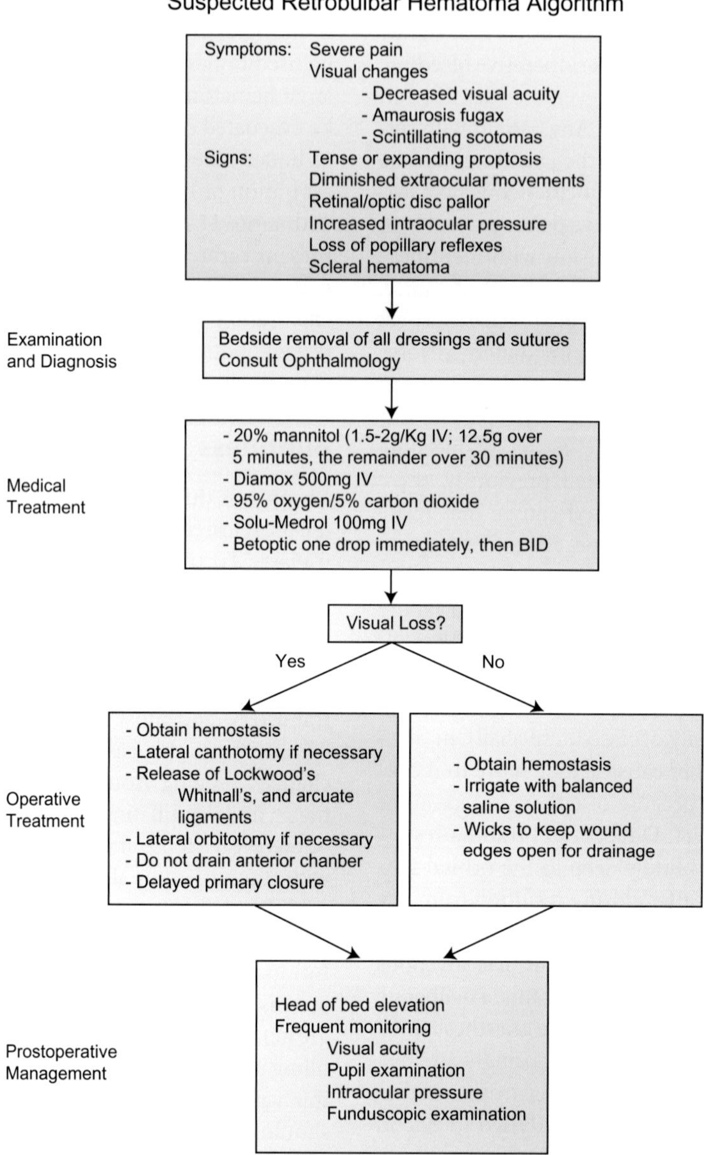

Figure 9-3. Algorithm for retrobulbar hematoma diagnosis and treatment. (From Rohrich RJ. Concepts in aesthetic upper blepharoplasty. Plast Reconstr Surg 2004;113:3.)

such as Betoptic (timolol; Allen USA, Fort Worth, TX) are also given. Carbogen (95% oxygen/5% carbon dioxide) can be administered to dilate the intraocular vessels. All these maneuvers should be employed in anticipation of returning to the operating room for re-exploration and evacuation of the hematoma. If no rapid improvement in symptoms occurs despite these measures, surgical intervention via a lateral canthotomy with inferior cantholysis is performed. Blindness is a rare, but catastrophic, complication and so the surgeon must be prepared to react to such a situation.

Chemosis

Almost every patient experiences some degree of bleeding, skin edema, and ecchymosis. Conjunctival chemosis, which is defined as a transudative edema of the bulbar and fornical conjunctiva, is characterized by visible swelling of the conjunctiva. This complication may occur in upper or lower blepharoplasty and may be transient, lasting 7–10 days, or severe, taking 2–5 months to resolve. Conjunctival inflammation is frequently present, in addition to epiphora, irritation, foreign body sensation, and

TABLE 9-3 Classification of Chemosis

Class	*Edema*	*Inflammation*	*Color*	*Lagophthalmos*	*Duration*
Type 1 (acute mild)	Mild	Mild	Yellow and/or pink	Absent	<3 wk
Type 2 (acute severe)	Severe	Severe	Yellow and/or pink	Present laterally (chemosis hinders closure	<3 wk
Type 3 (subchronic)	Mild to severe	Chronic	Pink	Absent	>3 wk–6 mo
Type 4 (subchronic because of lower lid malposition)	Severe	Moderate to severe	Pink	Lower lid malposition and/or ectropion	Until lid malposition is corrected

even visual alterations. Chemosis, however, more commonly occurs in lower lid blepharoplasty and is believed to result from blockage of orbital or eyelid lymphatics, exposure of the conjunctiva from lagophthalmos, regional edema, and excessive cautery during surgery. Weinfeld and coworkers suggested a classification of chemosis based on four general patterns of presentation: type 1, acute mild chemosis with complete lid closure; type 2, acute severe chemosis that prohibits complete lid closure; type 3, subchronic chemosis that persists longer than 3 weeks; and type 4, chemosis associated with eyelid malposition (**Table 9-3**). This situation, if persistent, can present a very frustrating problem for both the patient and the surgeon.

Several interventions have been suggested to prevent or reduce the occurrence of chemosis. Preoperative discontinuation of medications that may increase the risk of bleeding as well as a salt-restricted diet may minimize these events. Intraoperative measures include gentle handling of tissues during surgery, employing normotensive anesthesia, minimal use of intravenous fluids, and use of a tarsorrhaphy suture. Furthermore, the use of laser or radiofrequency incisional tools may further minimize ecchymosis, chemosis, and bleeding. Application of ice compresses for the first 24–48 hours postoperatively helps minimize edema and inflammation and makes patients more comfortable. Herbal preparations such as *Arnica Montana* have gained popularity over recent years as a remedy that decreases bruising, chemosis, and pain in the postoperative aesthetic patient. The true mechanism of action is not clear, but its effectiveness is at least measurable. Other therapies for chemosis and edema involve treatments directed at improving lymphatic drainage. Massage therapy for this purpose can be employed postoperatively to facilitate drainage and should be performed by a trained professional. Results are typically noted immediately and improve with daily sessions (**Figure 9-4**).

In most cases, chemosis resolves spontaneously early in the postoperative period, but for some patients, resolution is delayed. In such cases, a

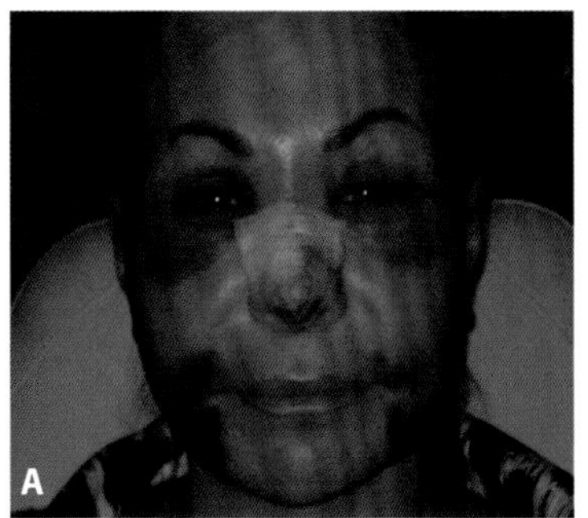

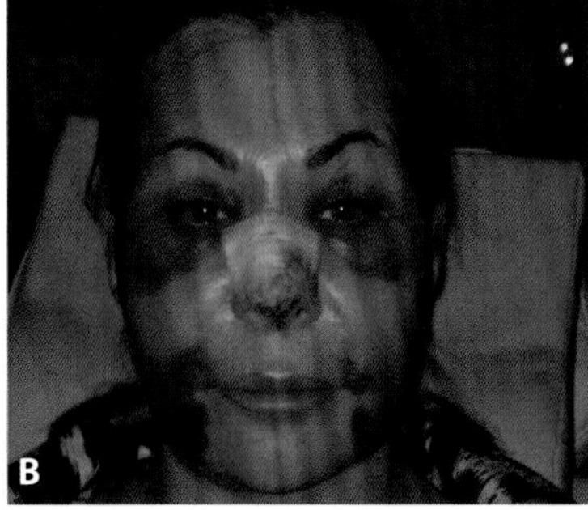

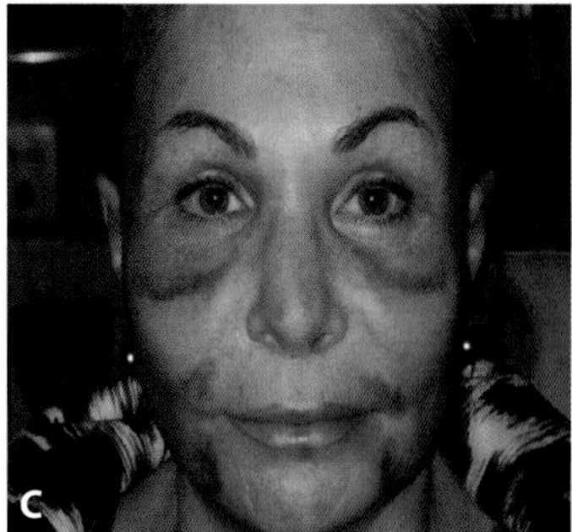

Figure 9-4 . (A-C) This 55-year-old woman had an endoscopic browlift, bilateral revision lower lid blepharoplasty, an endoscopic midface lift, and a revision rhinoplasty. (A) The patient 24 hours after surgery. (B) The same patient immediately after lymphatic drainage treatment with massage. Note the immediate changes in her eyes as the edema and chemosis improved. (C) The same patient 5 days after treatment.

treatment algorithm is followed in which the liberal use of wetting drops during the day and lubricating ophthalmic ointment at night is employed. If type 2 chemosis persists after 1 week, ocular decongestants like 2.5% Neo-Synephrine (Sanofi-Sythelabo, Inc., New York) and Tobradex (Alcon Laboratories, Inc., Fort Worth, TX) drops and ointment are used. Treatment is escalated if resolution has not occurred by the second postoperative visit by employing second-line steroids like FML Forte Liquifilm 0.25% (Allergan, Inc., Irvine, CA) or Pred Forte (Allergan). In some cases, the eye may be patched and even wrapped circumferentially with an elastic head wrap to provide mechanical pressure to downgrade and resolve the chemosis. If chemosis persists beyond 2 weeks and especially if significant lagophthalmos is present, surgical conjunctivotomy with possible tarsorrhaphy can be performed. Finally, oral steroids may be used for more severe cases or cases that have not been resolved by the aforementioned interventions.

Ocular Irritation/Dry Eye Syndrome

Patients can present with ocular irritation from several causes including dry eye syndrome, blepharitis, and alterations in the tear film and/or blink reflex. Dry eye syndrome affects up to 20% of women and 12% of men in the general population, and so it is critical to diagnose and treat this condition appropriately before surgery because the incidence of dry eye syndrome following blepharoplasty is between 8% and 21%. Ocular surface lubrication can be influenced by quantitative deficiencies such as decreased tear production, quality of the mucus and lipid layers of the tear film, and tear distribution problems secondary to a poor blink mechanism or from a combination of all these factors. Dry eye symptoms include discomfort, dryness, burning, stinging, foreign body sensation, gritty feeling, blurry vision, photophobia, itching, and redness.

Dry eye problems after blepharoplasty can be due to a number of factors. It is not uncommon for patients to have varying degrees of dry eye symptoms in the early postoperative period. These problems may be due to edema, which could interfere with the normal tear production and release. Fortunately, these symptoms improve and resolve after a short period. If persistent, however, the problem could have stemmed from a preexisting condition or a surgical complication. Risk factors for dry eyes include underlying systemic disease, menopause, previous eyelid surgery, and history of laser-assisted in situ keratileusis (LASIK). The preexisting conditions could be obvious and, in some cases, could be occult. As such, a thorough preoperative history and physical examination are of significant importance in preventing a postoperative dry eye syndrome. Symptoms such as foreign body sensation, burning, pain, and even lack of tearing should trigger the surgeons' need to further investigate. Sjögren's syndrome, rheumatoid arthritis, or systemic lupus erythromatosis and medications such as antihypertensives may decrease aqueous tear production and, as a result, may cause dry eye symptoms. A careful eye examination to include a Schirmer test is very helpful in predicting postoperative dry eye syndrome. This examination is capable of characterizing each of the components of the tear film. To perform this test, a Basic and a reflex (also known as a stimulated Schirmer test) is performed by placing a Schirmer test strip into the unanesthetized lower fornix, then measuring the length the tear travels after 5 minutes. A travel distance of 10 mm or more is normal, 5–10 mm is borderline, and less than 5 mm is abnormal. Although the results of Schirmer testing may be inconsistent, the test is beneficial for identifying severe dry eyes. In very severe cases, this may even be a contraindication to performing surgery. Drenser and colleagues identified that, by preserving the orbicularis muscle and its innervation, blepharoplasty could be performed safely in patients with dry eyes. Furthermore, preservation of the pretarsal orbicularis was cited as important even in patients without dry eye syndrome. The pumping action of this muscle is important in maintaining a uniform distribution of tears from blinking and clearance of the tears into the lacrimal drainage system. In addition to the aforementioned causes, postoperatively, lagophthalmos, lid malposition, and incomplete eye closure may all contribute to feeling of dry eyes.

The issue of LASIK surgery deserves special attention. Patients seeking cosmetic blepharoplasty generally fall within the age group of patients who are interested in undergoing LASIK surgery. With such patients, it is important to emphasize the increased risk of postoperative dry eye syndrome. Patients who undergo LASIK surgery alone have a 15%–25% chance of developing dry eye syndrome from a transient neurotropic keratopathy secondary to severing of the corneal sensory nerves during the surgery. Although these nerves tend to regenerate, the depth of ablation with LASIK surgery can increase the distance for regeneration and, as a result, the time to regenerate. This is relevant in the blepharoplasty patient because the normal corneal reflex that stimulates a blink reflex to sweep the cornea with tears is interrupted. Owing to the decreased corneal sensitivity, the blink is not elicited, and as a result, the tear film is not released. Furthermore, owing to the decreased sensation, the patient may not be aware of impending keratitis. Patients without a normal Bell's phenomenon could experience disastrous consequences. Michaeli and associates found evidence of decreased corneal sensitivity and tear production via Schirmer testing following LASIK, which resolved to normal levels after 3 months. Although there is no consensus as to the suggested timing of cosmetic surgery after LASIK, it is prudent that the cosmetic surgeon obtain a qualified evaluation of such patients prior to performing cosmetic blepharoplasty.

The treatment of preexisting ocular surface problems includes medical and surgical interventions. Medical therapies include lubrication with artificial tears or ointments, topical steroids, nonsteroidal anti-inflammatory drugs (NSAIDs), topical cyclosporine, and collagen/silicone punctual plugs. If the patient has blepharitis or meibomitis, the use of doxycycline, flax seed oil, omega-3 fatty acids, and warm compresses may help. Other preexisting conditions mentioned earlier, such as lid malposition, may be corrected during the surgical procedure. In summary, early recognition and treatment with eye lubrication is important, whereas addressing anatomical predisposing problems surgically is critical.

Corneal abrasion or injury to the globe is one of the most common, yet avoidable, complications of blepharoplasty. These can occur without diligent caution during the procedure. This is especially true when the patient is under general anesthesia and cannot respond to a stimulus. To prevent inadvertent injuries, instruments should not be passed over the eyes during surgery. If needed, corneal protectors may be used during blepharoplasty for added security, especially during training of resident surgeons. Alternatively, corneal protection may be achieved without using a corneal protector by maintaining eye closure during upper lid blepharoplasty. Transconjunctival lower blepharoplasty, however, puts the cornea at increased risk. In this case, everting the conjunctiva over the cornea with a 5.0 Prolene suture after the initial incision is made may protect the cornea. This maneuver also provides an added benefit of countertraction to increase the intraoperative exposure of the lower fat pads. Patients with severe eye pain and photophobia should be referred to an ophthalmologist for evaluation and treatment. Such patients with corneal abrasion may require ophthalmic antibiotics, steroids, and in some cases, an eye patch.

Application of scrub solution to the cornea has potentially disastrous effects. Use of chemicals such as chlorhexidine should be avoided altogether in the face because hydrolysis of the cornea and subsequent visual loss or blindness may occur. Gentler agents such as a dilute form of povidone-iodine solution or Technicare (Care-Tech Laboratories, Inc., St. Louis, MO) are safer around the eyes. Better yet, a protective coating of ophthalmic ointment or viscous tears could be placed in the eye prior to prepping the eye for surgery. In all cases, direct and deliberate placement of any prepping solution in the eye is strongly discouraged. If noted, the eye should be thoroughly irrigated with balanced saline solution (BSS) and monitored postoperatively for irritation. Minor abrasions may be treated with conservative therapy such as antibiotic ointments. Consultation with an ophthalmologist is strongly advised in all cases of injury to the globe. This is especially true with patients who complain of eye pain after surgery. Fortunately, more serious penetrating globe injuries during blepharoplasty are rare. Inadvertent injection of local anesthetic into the globe can occur. Such an injection can lead to a selective parasympathetic palsy, heralded by a fixed dilated pupil. If sufficient volume is injected, proptosis and increased intraocular pressure might result. In such cases, an immediate intraoperative urgent ophthalmology consult is necessary to exclude other ophthalmologic emergencies. Also, the measures outlined previously for treatment of retrobulbar hematoma may be warranted.

Suture Line and Wound Healing Complications

Suture line complications may include milia, inclusion cysts, and suture granuloma. Milia and inclusion cysts are common lesions that result from trapped epithelial debris beneath the healed skin surface or possibly from the occlusion of a glandular duct. They are typically associated with simple and running cuticular stitches. Their formation is minimized by subcuticular closure. Most of these problems are minor but may be very irritating to the patient. Each of these may be treated with observation or a minor procedure in the clinic to marsupialize or excise the inciting factor. This is done by using a no. 11 blade or 18-gauge needle to unroof the lesion and tease out the sac. Granulomas may develop as nodular thickenings within or beneath the suture line and are typically treated by steroid injections if small or by direct excision if large. Suture tunnels develop as a result of prolonged suture retention and epithelial surface migration along the suture tract. To prevent these suture tunnels from forming, early suture removal is encouraged (perhaps within 3–5 days). If tunnels develop, definitive treatment involves unroofing the tunnel. Suture marks are also related to the prolonged suture retention, and their formation can be avoided by using rapidly absorbing suture (fast-absorbing gut or mild chromic), by removing a monofilament suture early, or by employing subcuticular closure. Certain patients, however, may develop extreme erythema and edema in reaction to rapidly absorbing suture. This unpleasant occurrence is temporary but may require a significant amount of hand-holding and reassurance to the patient.

As the population of patients seeking cosmetic surgery evolves to include patients with darker skin, hypertrophic or prominent eyelid scars are becoming more common. Keloid scar formation has yet to be described in this region because the midface, lips, and periocular complex typically do not develop such lesions. However, hypertrophic scars are thought to develop owing to improper placement of lower and upper lid incisions. If extended too far medially in the epicanthal region, bowstring or web formation may occur. Extending the incisions to nasal skin should be avoided altogether because the nasal skin is thicker and has a different character. Should these scars develop, a Z-plasty can be performed to correct the deformity. A lateral canthal extension, which normally overlies the bony orbital rim prominence, that is oriented too obliquely downward or is closed under excessive tension predisposes an incision to hypertrophic scarring. If skin excision is performed as in a skin-muscle technique with associated midface lift and extended blepharoplasty, the difference in lower lid and lateral orbital skin thickness could lead to unwanted hypertrophic scarring that becomes noticeable, especially in men who typically do not use makeup. Proper execution of the procedure is the best way to prevent this problem, while also placing deep sutures to release tension off the skin closure.

Wound dehiscence may develop as a result of closure under tension, early removal of sutures, extension of a rare infectious process, or more commonly, hematoma. This phenomenon is seen more often in the lateral aspect of the incision with the skin-muscle and skin techniques. Treatment is directed to supportive taping or resuturing. If tension is too great for conservative management, then a lid suspension and lateral grafting, if necessary, is used. Skin slough may also develop as a result of devascularization of a skin segment. Typically, these problems are associated with hematoma formation. These hematomas must be evacuated, line of demarcation established, and appropriate skin replacement executed.

The risk of postoperative infection following periocular surgery altogether is very low, owing to the rich vascular supply of the eyelids. Nonetheless, one should obtain a history of shingles or herpes zoster virus because the stress of surgery could activate the quiescent virus, causing an outbreak with possible secondary infection. Such patients eliciting this history should be placed on prophylactic antiviral agents. Carter and coworkers reported the infection rate at 0.2% in patients who had undergone upper and lower blepharoplasty without laser resurfacing and slightly higher at 0.4% with laser resurfacing in addition to blepharoplasty. No studies have outlined the infection rate in patients in whom lasers have been used as an incision tool. Postoperative infections typically present between 4 and 7 days after surgery. Routine topical ophthalmic antibiotics are sufficient to treat these patients, with oral antibiotics and antiviral agents reserved for relatively immunocompromised (diabetic patients) or the aforementioned patients with shingles.

Upper Eyelid Complications

Complications of upper eyelid surgery generally occur as a result of improper planning, inadequate evaluation and improper preoperative marking, and surgical execution. An evaluation of the dynamics between the forehead, the brows, and the upper eyelids is critical in determining the extent of excess upper lid skin or the true diagnosis of the problem needing surgical attention. Furthermore, a clear distinction must be made between true eyelid ptosis, brow ptosis, blepharochalasis, and dermatochalasis or a true upper eyelid skin excess. This is important because the patient seeking rejuvenation of the eyes typically complains of the tired look suggesting upper eyelid problems or the unhappy appearance typically pertaining to the brow. Moreover, these

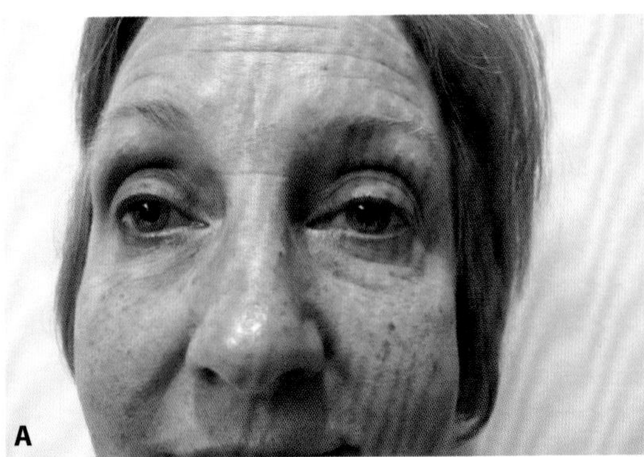

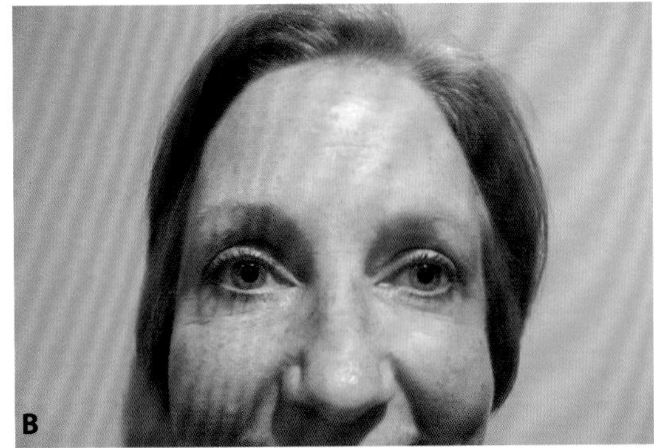

Figure 9-5. (A) This patient has a combination of brow ptosis with senile levator dysfunction leading to ptosis. Careful evaluation of the patient led to the appropriate procedures performed including a browlift and upper lid blepharoplasty with ptosis repair (and lower lid fat sculpture). (B) Her postoperative photo reveals a significant improvement and a more youthful appearance

findings could occur in isolation or in combination and, as such, must be recognized in order to perform the appropriate procedure (**Figure 9-5**). Blepharochalasis is a recurrent, intermittent inflammatory condition of the eyelids resulting in edema, erythema, and thin excess eyelid skin secondary to histamine response and related to increased immunoglobulin E levels. This condition is felt to have a genetic component and is typically seen in younger patients. In contrast to dermatochalasis, blepharochalasis is difficult to correct and likely to recur. This condition must be distinguished from dermatochalasis, which represents a true excess of upper eyelid skin that has lost elasticity and support due to aging.

The position of the eyelid crease is perhaps the most important landmark for the upper lid blepharoplasty. As such, preoperative markings are critical to assess and are made with the nonsedated patient sitting upright in neutral gaze. The brow needs to be elevated to the proper position before marks are made. The incision is usually hidden in the supratarsal fold formed by the upper eyelid crease. This fold is located at approximately 8–10 mm above the ciliary margin in women and at 7–8 mm in men. The upper marking is typically made at least 10 mm from the lower edge of the brow and not to include any thick brow skin. Typically, one is able to see a distinct difference in color from the upper lid skin and the brow. This color difference can assist the surgeon in delineating the limits of the upper eyelid excision. The use of the pinch test for redraping the skin is also helpful. Typically, the shape of the skin resection is lenticular in younger patients and more trapezoid-shaped laterally in older patients due to the excess lateral hooding seen in older patients. The incisions may need to be extended laterally with a larger excision, but extension lateral to the orbital rim should be avoided if possible to prevent a prominent scar, especially in male patients who have thick skin and typically do not use makeup. Similarly, the medial markings should not extend medial to the medial canthus for larger resections because extensions onto the nasal sidewall may result in webbing. If excessive skin is present medially, a W-plasty may need to be performed. A high crease may be a sign of levator aponeurosis dehiscence and involutional ptosis. In that case, the eyelid crease must be marked lower to the existing crease. After repair of the ptosis, with advancement of the levator aponeurosis, the eyelid crease should be reformed at the desired level, taking small bites of the orbicularis muscle when closing the skin. Failure to recognize patients with a high crease, who actually do not have excessive upper lid skin, may lead to excessive skin excision and its associated symptoms. Also, the high crease in addition to the hollowed look could lead to a very dissatisfied patient.

Ptosis

Dehiscence of the levator aponeurosis, whether congenital, traumatic, senile (**Figure 9-6**), or iatrogenic, can present with ptosis of the upper eyelid. As such, a measurement of the intrapalpebral distance (typically between 10 and 12 mm) aids in distinguishing these phenomena. This measurement can further be divided into the mean reflex distance (MRD) 1 and 2. The MRD 1 (typically 2.5–5 mm) represents the distance from the center of the pupil up to the

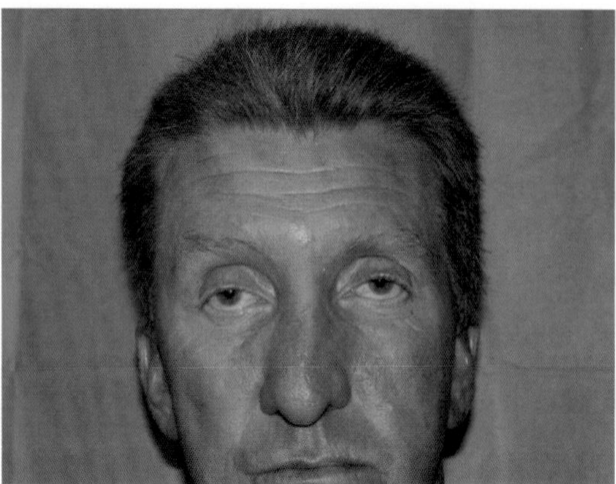

Figure 9-6. This patient presents with true senile levator dysfunction and, as a result, ptosis. His MRD-1 shows a marked abnormality. Also note his elevated palpebral fissure as well as compensation elevation of his brow.

inferior edge of the upper eyelid. The MRD 2 represents the distance from the center of the pupil down to the superior edge of the lower eyelid. So, a patient with eyelid ptosis will have an MRD 1, which is less than 2.5 mm. This finding should alert the surgeon that a blepharoplasty alone may not be the right intervention for the patient, and an evaluation by an ophthalmologist or oculoplastic surgeon may be necessary.

Ptosis of the eyelid deserves special attention because proper diagnosis and classification is very important in preventing complications relating to this phenomenon. Classifying ptosis according to time of onset as congenital or acquired is very useful for directing the choice of surgical procedure for repair. Ptosis can further be classified according to pathophysiology as aponeurotic, myogenic, neurogenic, mechanical, or pseudoptosis (**Table 9-4**).

TABLE 9-4 Classification of Ptosis

Aponeurogenic
Involutional
Ocular surgery
Contact lens wear
Trauma
Myogenic
Chronic progressive external ophthalmoplegia
Myasthenia gravis
Oculopharyngeal syndrome
Myotonic dystrophy
Trauma
Neurogenic
Third nerve palsy
Homer's syndrome
Trauma
Mechanical
Lid tumor
Cicatricial
Symblepharon
Trauma
Pseudoptosis
Enophthalmos
Microphthalmos
Hypotropia
Contralateral proptosis or lid retraction
Trauma

Aponeurogenic ptosis is the most common type of acquired ptosis and is most frequently associated with dermatochalasis. As such, the facial plastic surgeon is more likely to encounter such and should be astute in the evaluation process. Here, the levator muscle is normal, but the levator aponeurosis is attenuated or dehisced from its normal insertions on the tarsal plate and the orbicularis muscle. This type of ptosis is characterized by normal levator function and is usually accompanied by an elevated lid crease. It may be a naturally occurring involutional change or it may be precipitated by intraocular surgery, long-term daily contact lens wear, or trauma. Myogenic ptosis, conversely, is most commonly congenital and involves an abnormal levator muscle infiltrated with fibrous or adipose tissue. It is characterized by poor levator function due to maldevelopment of levator muscle fibers. Neurogenic ptosis results from interruption of normally developed innervations. Mechanical ptosis may be caused by any process that weighs down the eyelid, such as lid neoplasm, or any process that tethers the eyelid posteriorly. Finally, the surgeon should not be misled by pseudoptosis, a condition that creates an impression of ptosis when true ptosis does not exist. This can occur in cases of globe malposition such as enophthalmos, microphthalmos, or even thyroid orbitopathy where unilateral lid retraction presents the false impression of ptosis in the contralateral lid. Wherever suspected, the facial plastic surgeon is encouraged to obtain a formal consultation to the ophthalmologist for appropriate evaluation and documentation.

When ptosis is suspected, the contralateral eye must also be checked in patients with unilateral or asymmetrical ptosis to ascertain the presence or absence of Hering's law. Hering's law of equal innervations to agonist muscle proposes that the levator muscles of both upper eyelids are bilaterally and equally innervated. The attempt to elevate a ptotic lid results in excess innervations to that levator muscle and, consequently, to the contralateral levator muscle as well. This results in contralateral lid retraction and subsequent asymmetry. With the ptotic eye occluded, the examiner checks to see whether the MRD 1 decreases appreciably in the contralateral eye. This finding suggests that there is bilateral ptosis, consistent with Hering's law If undetected preoperatively, an unsuspected postoperative drop in the opposite eyelid will occur, leading to both patient and surgeon dissatisfaction. As such, if Hering's law is detected preoperatively, it may indicate the need for bilateral levator surgery in a patient with unilateral or asymmetrical ptosis. Failure to recognize these problems could result in the undesirable lagophthalmos and its problems, upper eyelid asymmetries, and the unhappy patient.

The levator excursion is perhaps the best clinical test for levator function. This measures the distance between extreme upward gaze and downward gaze, with the brow immobilized in the neutral position with the examiner's thumb, eliminating any contribution of the brow to lid elevation. Patients determined to have minimal ptosis require a stimulated test with phenylephrine in the involved eye. This is done by instilling 2.5% or 10% phenylephrine in the tested eye and then waiting 5 minutes. The MRD 1 is then checked in both eyes. A rise in the MRD 1 of 1.5 mm is considered a positive test indicating that Muller's muscle is intact and viable.

New postoperative ptosis reflects levator muscle or aponeurosis injury intraoperatively and is noted when the upper eyelid margin covers the upper limbus by more than 2–3 mm while on neutral gaze. This problem typically occurs with upper blepharoplasty techniques that involve the invagination of upper eyelid skin by levator aponeurosis imbrications. With the traditional skin-muscle technique practiced by most facial plastic surgeons, injury to the aponeurosis can still occur. The most common cause is excision of the orbicularis oculi muscle near the pretarsal area, with poorly developed or identified planes of dissection. This is adjacent to the area where the levator inserts on to the tarsus. Another cause of injury is direct injury to the tarsus itself, with accompanying tarsal hematoma and compromise of the levator insertion. If injury is recognized intraoperatively, it should be repaired immediately using permanent braided sutures or polydioxanone suture (PDS). Intraoperative consultation to an oculoplastic surgeon may be obtained if the surgeon feels less comfortable with this intervention. Postoperatively, levator aponeurosis disinsertion is diagnosed by the presence of ptosis, a thin upper eyelid, and a high upper eyelid fold, in the face of retained full eyelid excursion. It is graded as mild (1–2 mm of ptosis), moderate (2–3 mm), or severe (> 4 mm). Repair of the injured levator aponeurosis is mandatory for good recovery and should be performed by a surgeon skilled in ptosis repair. Consultation with an oculoplastic surgeon is advised.

Lagophthalmos

Lagophthalmos or incomplete upper eyelid closure is a normal occurrence in the early postoperative period. This usually resolves within 48 hours of the operation and is caused by eyelid edema and intraoperative anesthetic infiltration. Intraoperatively, up to 3 mm of lagophthalmos is acceptable in the sedated patient or the patient under general anesthesia. However, early postoperative or intraoperative lagophthalmos greater than 4 mm or any persistent lagophthalmos indicates overexcision of upper lid skin. If recognized, the treatment of choice is grafting of the excised skin because it provides the best possible match for color and thickness. If suspected, the excised skin is retained refrigerated in normal saline for up to 3 weeks, giving ample time for resolution of postoperative edema, while still having an excellent rate of survival as a full-thickness skin graft. If left untreated, lagophthalmos could lead to severe dry eye symptoms including chemosis, corneal exposure, and tearing. Fortunately, eyelid massage and observation resolve most occurrences of lagophthalmos. Nonetheless, conservative excision and meticulous preoperative evaluation are paramount in preventing lagophthalmos.

Asymmetry

Careful identification of preexisting asymmetries is very important in preventing an unhappy patient postoperatively. These preexisting asymmetries of the brows or upper eyelids are the most common causes of postoperative asymmetries of the upper eyelid. After aesthetic blepharoplasty, patients typically inspect the work of the surgeon in detail, identifying every discrepancy, even those that could have been present preoperatively. Thus, during the preoperative evaluation and discussion, the wise surgeon will carefully reveal these existing asymmetries in every patient and point them out. The

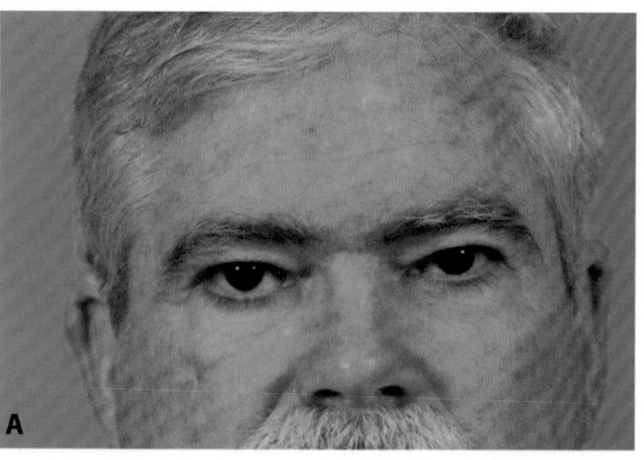

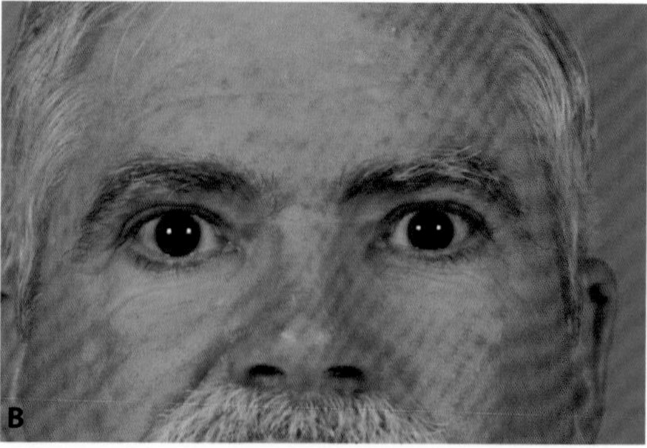

Figure 9-7. (A and B) Pre- and postoperative photos of a male with brow asymmetry and significant upper lid dermatochalasis. He had an endobrow lift and bilateral upper lid blepharoplasty. His asymmetry was not fully corrected, but the very satisfied patient was counseled appropriately and recognized the preexisting asymmetry

informed patient will credit the surgeon as very astute and observant, rather than inattentive and imprecise if the asymmetry is not mentioned until after the fact (**Figure 9-7**). In the immediate postoperative period, small asymmetries frequently occur during healing but improve with time.

Brow position is an important determinant of eyelid position where an asymmetrical brow leads to preoperative asymmetrical dermatochalasis. Attention should also be directed to noting any evidence of deep superior sulcus because the degree of depth of the superior sulcus is determined by the interplay between the brow fat, the preaponeurotic fat pads, the orbital septum, and the levator aponeurosis. In severe brow asymmetries, it is prudent to correct this asymmetry with a brow lift followed by a blepharoplasty either simultaneously or several weeks later. Correction of asymmetries should be performed only following a detailed discussion with the patient, because these can change the patient's natural expression. Also, care must be taken to differentiate passive asymmetries from dynamic asymmetries because dynamic asymmetries must not be corrected. If performed simultaneously, meticulous preoperative marking is very helpful. Here, the awake, nonsedated patient is placed in a sitting position and the brow is manually elevated to the desired position, keeping in mind the inherent asymmetry while the desired excision of eyelid skin is delineated. The young inexperienced surgeon is advised to perform the brow lift and blepharoplasty at separate times, typically several weeks apart.

Pseudo fat herniation is evaluated preoperatively by physical examination and photos. One of the most common complications of blepharoplasty is the asymmetry caused by excision of fat. The amount of fat to be excised should ideally be determined preoperatively, with the patient in upgaze, downgaze, and medial and lateral ranges of motion, with photographic documentation. The excision of fat then must be guided by marking, meticulous injection, and availability of these photographs intraoperatively. The amount excised should be enough only to provide improved cosmesis. This is done by excising the fat that "comes naturally to you" and not that which you have to aggressively tease out. Excessive excision can lead to asymmetry and, worse, the hollow look that is so undesirable. The fat from each compartment is saved on the back table on marked sheets of gauze that delineate their source and compared at the end of the case. If asymmetries are noted at this time, re-implantation of fat as a free graft can be performed to camouflage the asymmetry. If, however, the imperfection goes unnoticed until after the surgery, and the cosmetic result is suboptimal, autogenous fat may be implanted as a revision procedure.

Complications of the Lower Lid

Lower eyelid blepharoplasty is a very commonly performed procedure designed to reduce dermatochalasis and pseudoherniated fat from the lower eyelid. When performed successfully, this procedure significantly enhances the youthfulness of the eyes. Unfortunately, blepharoplasty of the lower eyelid is among the most challenging operations in facial plastic surgery because there are several potential pitfalls in the execution of this procedure. As mentioned earlier in the chapter, the lower eyelid is divided anatomically into the anterior, middle, and posterior lamella. The anterior lamella includes skin and orbicularis muscle. The middle lamella includes the orbital septum, attached at the arcus marginalis on the bony rim and superiorly to the inferior eyelid retractors. The posterior lamella includes inferior retractor muscles (capsulopalpebral fascia and inferior tarsal muscle), tarsus, and palpebral conjunctiva. These lamellae are intimately associated, and their interactions contribute to the contour and position of the lower eyelid. During the aging process, the lower eyelid–cheek junction develops an uneven contour secondary to descent of the cheek, with increased prominence of the lower lid fat, resulting in a nasojugal groove with a tear trough deformity. Patients seeking cosmetic lower eyelid rejuvenation should be evaluated for evidence of eyelid malposition, descent of the malar fat pads, poor maxillary bony support, stretching of the lateral canthal tendons, poor tearing, corneal exposure, eyelid retraction, lower lid hollowing, scleral show, and lid laxity. A thorough knowledge of the anatomy of the lower eyelid and the aesthetic relationships of the lower lid to the midface are critical to performing the appropriate surgery and thus preventing complications. Lower eyelid malposition, asymmetries in fat distribution, and diplopia are difficult complications that, unfortunately, do occur in more frequency than earlier thought.

Lower Eyelid Malposition

Malposition of the lower eyelid is a common, yet undesirable, complication reported in 10%–20% of lower eyelid blepharoplasties. It is a general term that can present as a spectrum of more defined problems ranging from lateral rounding and scleral show to lid retraction and cicatricial ectropion. Appropriate position of the lower lid is defined when the lower lid margin is at the level of the inferior limbus and the tarsus is approximated against the globe. A good estimation of this ideal position can be made by measuring the MRD 2, which is defined as the distance from the light reflex reflected from the cornea when the eye is in primary gaze to the lower eyelid margin. Malposition occurs when the eyelid is deviated from this ideal position (**Figure 9-8**). The term scleral show refers to the findings of increased white sclera when the lid is below its ideal position. This condition may occur naturally and may tip the surgeon as to the presence of senile lid laxity. Iatrogenic scleral show, however, typically occurs laterally, although there may be scleral show on the nasal or middle of the lid margin, exposing a weak medial canthal tendon.

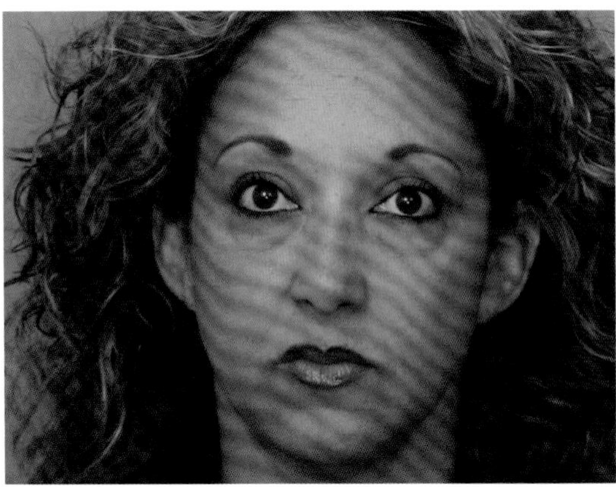

Figure 9-8. This patient illustrates malposition of the lower eyelids with her right eye worse than the left. The normal position of her lower eyelid should be at the lower limbus.

A careful examination of the lower eyelid includes assessment for degree of lower lid laxity. Assessment of lid supporting structures can be done via the lid distraction test and the lid retraction or snap back test. A lid distraction test (**Figure 9-9**) is performed by gently grasping the lower lid and distracting it out anteriorly. The lid is considered lax if it can be distracted greater than 8–10 mm. A lid retraction test (**Figure 9-10**), which assesses the function of the orbicularis muscle and the amount of lid tone, is performed by retracting the lower eyelid vertically and allowing it to "snap" back into position. A fast snap of the lower eyelid to the proper position indicates normal tension. Conversely, laxity is considered mild, with simply a slow return to normal position, or more severe, in which normal position is not returned without excessive blinking or assistance into position. Adjunctive maneuvers and

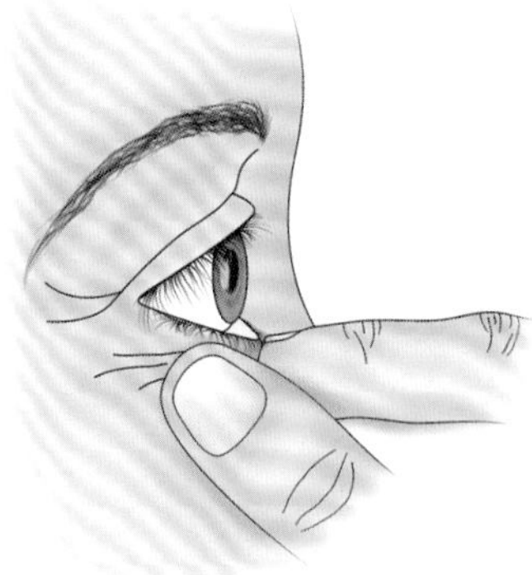

Figure 9-9. Lid distraction test used to assess laxity of tarsoligamentous sling.

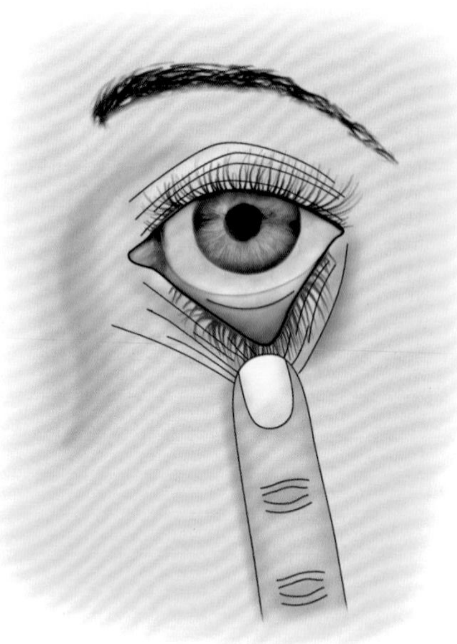

Figure 9-10. Lid retraction test used to assess lower eyelid tone and stability of medial and lateral canthal tendon attachments.

procedures may minimize chances for lid malposition due to lid laxity. Horizontal tightening procedures include simple lateral canthal placation, wedge excision, lateral tarsal strip, and even lateral canthal repositioning procedures. Details of the indications and technical details are beyond the scope of this chapter. When considering lower lid tightening, the surgeon must beware of the patient with the "negative vector" lower lid. For this reason, the patient also should be assessed in the lateral position to determine the relative globe position. A prominent globe and recessed orbital rim predispose the patient to the potential for postoperative malposition. This relationship is described as the "negative vector" in that the line drawn from the midpupil to the bony orbital rim on the lateral view falls backward from superior to inferior (**Figures 9-11 and 9-12**). If the lower lid is tightened in this situation, the lid may actually assume a worsened or lower position akin to an obese man's belt slipping further down his belly when the belt is cinched tighter. As such, the mnemonic "big eyes, big trouble" is relevant and should be heeded by the facial plastic surgeon. In patients with the negative vector, midfacial augmentation may be the intervention of choice, rather than the lower lid blepharoplasty that the patient perhaps requested. Undoing an ill-advised blepharoplasty in such patients is one of the most difficult endeavors in facial plastic surgery (**Figure 9-13**). Other perioperative maneuvers may also reduce the risk of lid malposition. Various authors have described the use of an orbicularis suspension suture when performing a transcutaneous approach. This stitch suspends the lateral orbicularis to the inner part of the lateral orbital rim, thereby reducing tension on closure in the subciliary area. Other maneuvers may include temporary tarsorrhaphy or a Frost suspension stitch to the lateral brow and simple taping of the lower lid superiorly and laterally. Early recognition of lid malposition and intervention with these rather benign maneuvers may reverse the problem before it becomes a long-term issue. In all, after careful assessment of the patients' physical findings, the type of lower blepharoplasty the surgeon chooses and the technical details of the procedure can have a significant effect on eyelid position for the patient.

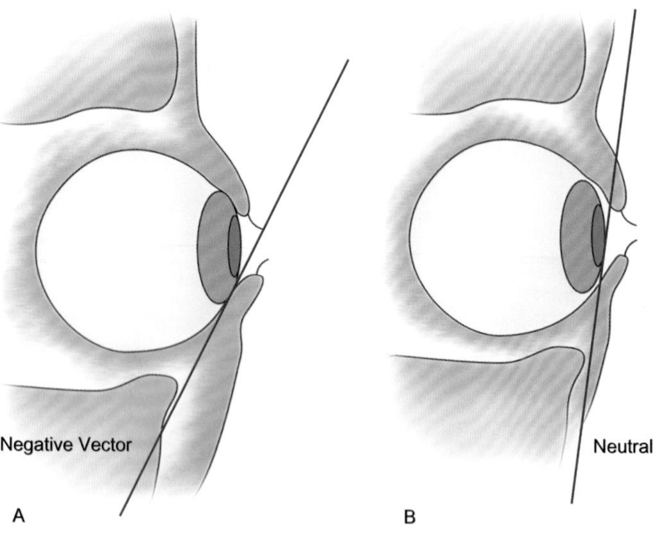

Figure 9-11. (A) The "negative vector." A line from the globe to the inferior orbital rim is drawn on the lateral view, and if the line falls from an anterosuperior posteroinferior inclination, a negative vector is present. This condition is attributed to the globe that rests anterior to the orbital rim shelf. (B) A more "neutral vector" that is a safer configuration for lower eyelid surgery.

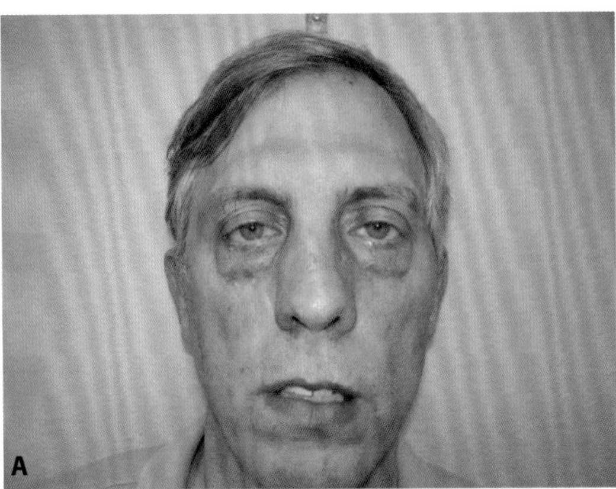

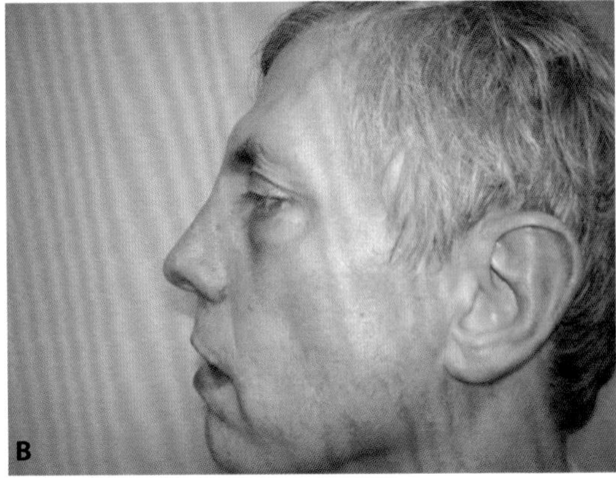

Figure 9-12. (A and B) This patient has a "negative vector." His globe rests anterior to the orbital rim shelf. The mnemonic "big eyes, big trouble" recalls the danger of operating on these patients because performing a lower lid tightening procedure may further exacerbate the problem. Note that, in this patient, he also has lateral scleral show, which may be exacerbated by any form of surgery

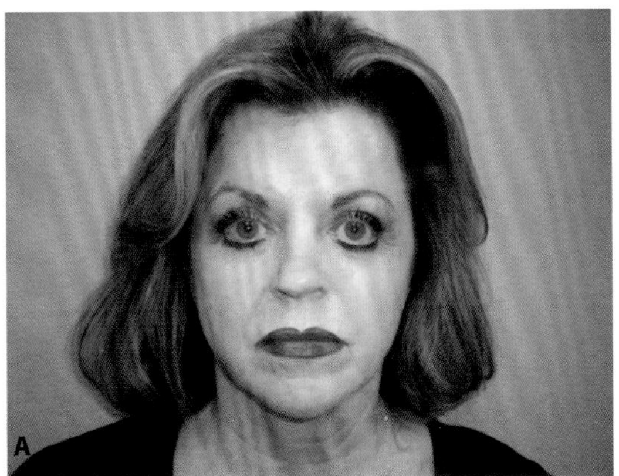

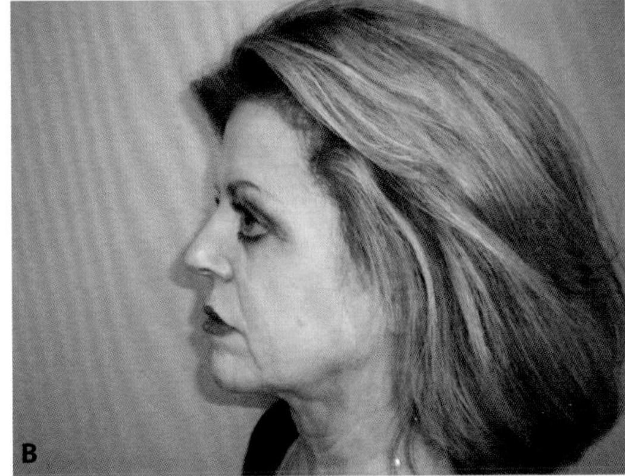

Figure 9-13. (A and B) A patient with a "negative vector" who had a lower lid blepharoplasty with attempts at horizontal lid tightening procedures. Note her lateral scleral show with lid retraction. She refused lid reconstruction with palatal graft.

Eyelid malposition may be related to the technique chosen, which can influence the degree of lamellar disruption, degree of tissue excision, and laxity of the lower eyelid. Procedures that disrupt the anterior lamella, such as subcutaneous or skin-muscle flaps, place the patient at risk for ectropion. Procedures that disrupt the middle lamella include transeptal fat excision via a transcutaneous or transconjunctival, preseptal approach, septal tightening procedures with cautery, and trans-suborbicularis oculi fat midface lifts. All these may lead to lid retraction. Generally, transcutaneous blepharoplasties are associated with a higher incidence of this problem than transconjunctival approaches. The transconjunctival incision avoids the orbital septum and, therefore, minimizes the risks of lower eyelid retraction from middle lamellar inflammation/scarring. The other advantage of a transconjunctival incision is that the dynamics of eyelid closure, including tear pumping and tear distribution, are not affected with preservation of the orbicularis muscle and its innervations. Perkins and colleagues compared the indications, expected results, postoperative complications, and patient satisfaction in 300 successive cases of skin-muscle flap approach with cases in which the transconjunctival approach was used. In many cases, adjunctive procedures such as simultaneous chemical peeling and the "pinch" technique for redundant skin excision were employed. They found that both short- and long-term complications were significantly reduced with the transconjunctival approach as compared with the skin-muscle flap approach. McCollough and associates, conversely, reported excellent results with negligible incidence of unacceptable scar and eyelid malposition in a retrospective observational study involving 50 patients who had the transcutaneous skin-muscle flap approach to the lower eyelid. Regardless of the technique used, however, there is potential for lid malposition with any approach when the inappropriate forces take effect. Lid malposition has even been observed with some chemical or laser skin tightening techniques as well.

The causes of lower eyelid retraction are multifactorial. Lower eyelid malposition after cosmetic surgery may be due to inadequate skin (excessive excision of eyelid skin leading to anterior lamellar insufficiency), which could be associated with lower eyelid laxity due to lateral canthal tendon laxity or disinsertion. Deficiency of the anterior lamella due to previous surgery or trauma may be assessed on preoperative examination by having the patient look up with the mouth open. Typically, anterior lamellar insufficiency leads to cicatrical ectropion, which is a malposition in which the lower eyelid is everted away from the globe (**Figure 9-14**). This may present early, if the patient is symptomatic, or late, months or even years after the initial blepharoplasty when the presenting signs are more cosmetic and show the "operated" look. If the patient presents within a few months of the initial procedure, treatment options could include lyses of adhesions and a lid suspension procedure. Later, treatment of this type of lid malposition may include lower lid skin grafts and also midface lifting. Far less common is cicatricial entropion that presents as an inversion of the eyelid margin. This may be the result of a lid tightening procedure or scarring of the posterior lamella.

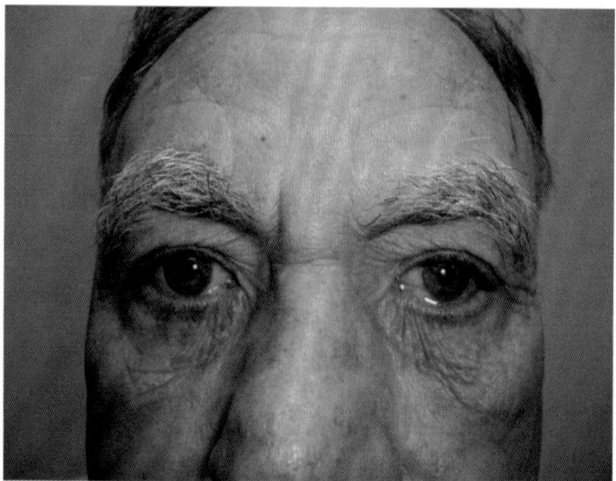

Figure 9-14. This 70-year-old man had bilateral lower lid blepharoplasties 20 years prior and subsequently developed bilateral ectropion with associated epiphora in his left eye that he attributed to allergies. Careful examination revealed an eversion of the punctum of the lacrimal duct away from the globe. Digital repositioning of the lid pleasantly resulted in resolution of his epiphora. Note the lateral scleral show and the tears pooled in his left eye.

Middle lamella inflammation and subsequent scarring may also occur singularly or in combination with anterior lamellar problems, as previously stated. In any case, the resultant contracture of the orbital septum will cause the lower eyelid to pull inferiorly from its normal position. Middle lamella scarring presenting as a late complication of cosmetic surgery appears with the lower eyelid vertically retracted but not pulled away from the eye, as seen in anterior lamella insufficiency. This condition has been attributed to inflammation of the fat pads, in which fat manipulation or resection is the initial inflammation-inciting event. The subsequent inflammation results in scarring, fibrosis, and contracture between the orbital septum anteriorly and the capsulopalpebral fascia posteriorly. As such, a single dense band of scar is formed, resulting in retraction (**Figure 9-15**). As the orbital septum fibroses and contracts, there is a resultant shortening of the distance between the inferior tarsal boarder and the orbital rim, where the orbital septum originates. This orbital septum scarring and fibrosis pulls the lower eyelid down closer to its origin on the anterior maxilla. The lower eyelid fat is then pushed posteriorly into the orbit by this scar, contributing to the hollow appearance seen in the lower eyelids and the distinct cheek-lid interface that is characteristic to patients with lid retraction after cosmetic surgery.

Understanding lower eyelid descent and its relationship with midface descent as well as the influence of cosmetic surgery on orbital septum/capsulopalpebral fascia scarring is very important. This knowledge is necessary to evaluate patients properly and to choose the appropriate surgical intervention to reposition the lower eyelids and midface back to their normal anatomic positions. Patipa described a methodical approach to the management of complications based on this knowledge and designed various techniques tailored to each patient. Initial conservative management of lower lid retraction, however, includes massage of the area of scarring and use of lubricating agents and even steroids. These maneuvers can be employed as soon as retraction is suspected, or indeed to prevent or control inflammation of the middle or posterior

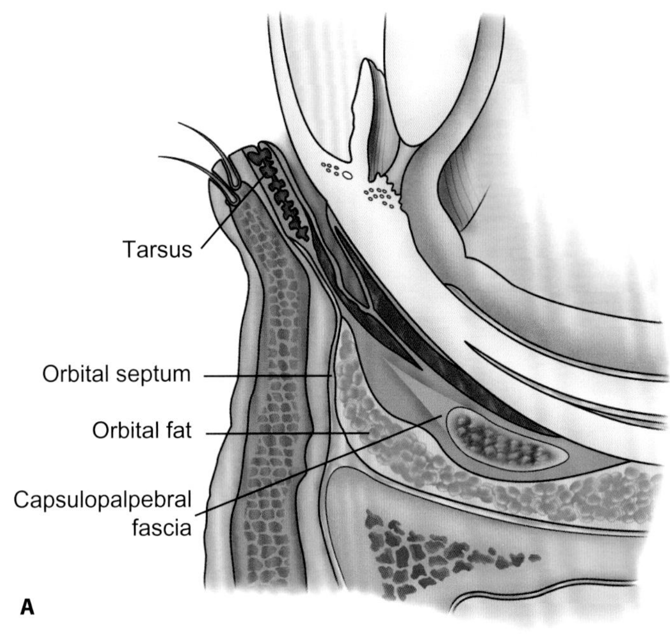

Figure 9-15. (A) Normal lower eyelid anatomy. Note the insertion of the orbital septum on the capsulopalpebral fascia. (B) Lower eyelid retraction. Note the scarring and fusion between the orbital septum and the capsulopalpebral fascia, which results in lower eyelid retraction and posterior displacement of the orbital fat. This contributes to the hollow-eyed appearance in these patients after cosmetic surgery.

lamella. Postoperative correction of lid malposition, after wounds have healed and the forces of scar contracture are in effect, is a far more difficult endeavor than preoperative avoidance. Nonetheless, the surgeon must be prepared to treat such conditions.

Anterior lamellar deficiencies due to excessive skin excision can be treated with a skin graft and lateral canthal tendon tightening procedure. In cases in which the patient has lower eyelid and midface malposition, the patient could undergo a lateral canthal tendon tightening procedure, placement of a mucosal graft spacer, and subperiosteal midface elevation. This recruits enough skin to avoid the need for skin grafts and repositions the

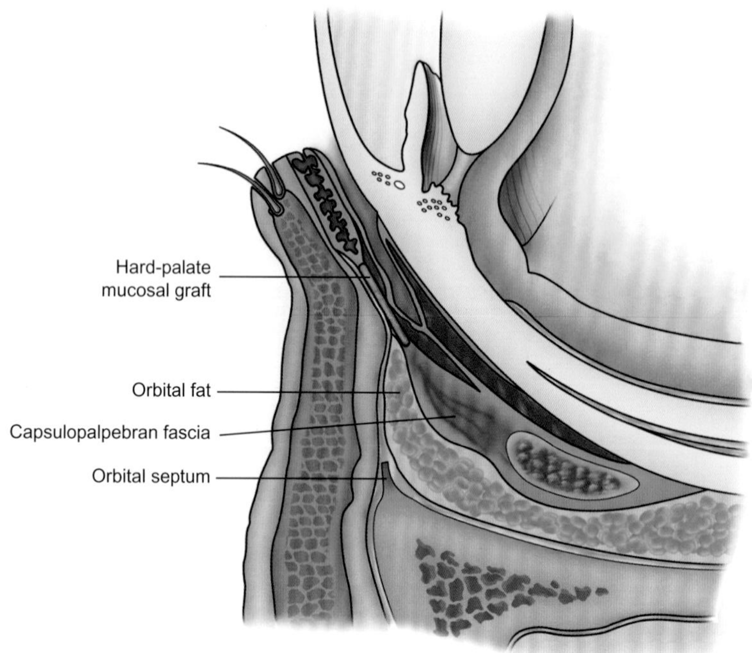

Figure 9-16. Illustration of capsulopalpebral fascia released from inferior tarsus and recessed, the inserted hard palate/mucosal graft spacer, and the released, scarred orbital septum. This allows orbital fat to return to its normal anatomic position.

lid and all midface structures back to their normal, anatomically favorable position. Posterior and middle lamellar contracture is more often treated with lysis of adhesions and placement of a spacer graft in the conjunctival area that will support the lid in position. Such graft options include hard palate, conchal skin, and cartilage composite grafts; free conchal cartilage grafts; acellular dermis; and other similar grafts (**Figure 9-16**). In summary, avoidance is the best way to minimize the complication of lower lid malposition through careful evaluation of the patient preoperatively and meticulous choice and execution of surgical intervention. Correcting problems with lid malposition also involves careful evaluation of the cause of the problem with prompt intervention before additional injury to the eye occurs. A detailed knowledge of the anatomy and the aging effects on the eyelid is critical to diagnosing the problems as well as avoiding the potential pitfalls. The surgeon who endeavors to perform such procedures is encouraged to have a solid grasp of these concepts.

Excessive Fat Excision

One of the hallmarks of the overcorrected aging eyelid is excessive excision of periorbital fat via a variety of approaches. The result may give the patient and appearance of hollowed-out or sunken eyes, an appearance that may be almost cadaveric. In such cases, the inferior orbital rim may be prominent (**Figure 9-17**) and, in most cases, is accentuated by descent of the malar fat pad or the SOOF. Such a look is counterintuitive to the philosophy that a youthful eye includes significant tissue volume. The result may be that patient looks aged and older. Blepharoplasty is no longer a procedure solely of tissue excision but is more now a return of the volume lost during aging as well as replacing the contour of youthfulness. Awareness of such concepts by the surgeon during a careful preoperative analysis may prevent overzealous fat resection. Modern adjuncts

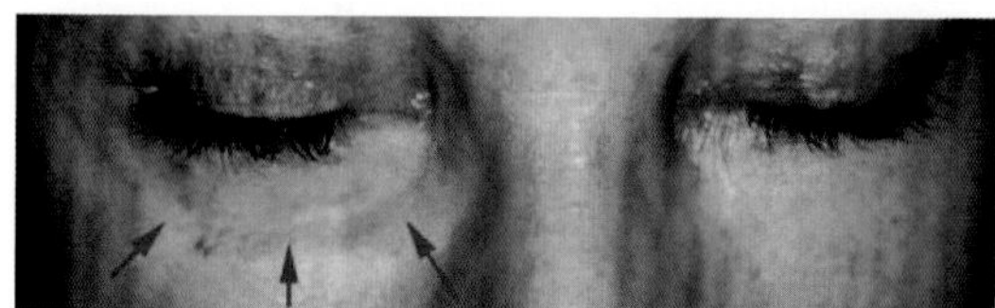

Figure 9-17. Patient with overaggressive periorbital fat excision. Note the prominent infraorbital rim as indicated by the *red arrows*. Correction with autologous fat injections or volume fillers would be needed to repair this complication.

to blepharoplasty include the use of volume fillers such a hyaluronic acid, dermal fat, and autologous fat transfer. Fat transposition from the orbit to the orbital rim is also used to fill the hollows of the aging lower eyelid tear trough and nasojugal folds. Tissue volume fillers are also options for correcting volume and contour irregularities that result after blepharoplasty. Particularly with transconjunctival procedures, where skin is not addressed, fat excision can also lead to redundancy of the lower eyelid skin. The surgeon must introduce this concept to the patient preoperatively and may augment the procedure with something to address the skin, such as a chemical or laser peel or even a simple skin pinch. Many surgeons who are well aware of problems associated with over-resection of fat may inadvertently under-resect fat as well and inadequately treat pseudo fat herniation. This may require a revision of the original procedure. Alternatively, the surgeon may consider camouflaging options with volume fillers as described previously.

Diplopia/Strabismus

Transient diplopia may occur as a result of local anesthesia or orbital edema. Injury to extraocular muscles, most commonly the inferior oblique muscle in lower blepharoplasty, may result in diplopia postoperatively. This is most often temporary, although significant trauma can be longer lasting, and consultation with an oculoplastic surgeon is imperative for definitive treatment. The risk of diplopia can be decreased during lower lid blepharoplasty by identifying and avoiding the inferior oblique muscle as it courses between the nasal and the central lower lid compartments. In addition, cautery should be judicious so as to not introduce excessive thermal injury to the muscles or nerves in the orbit. In addition, strabismus may occur secondary to restrictive changes from scar formation. Nonresolving diplopia following blepharoplasty may require strabismus surgery if the patient remains symptomatic.

Lateral Rounding

This complication should not be confused with lid malpositioning resulting in scleral show and other findings. Lateral rounding occurs as a result of scarring related to incision in this area. Typically, patients who may have had a lid tightening procedure develop blunting of the lateral canthal area, especially if the procedure is not performed meticulously or if inappropriate sutures are used. Another possible cause includes a subciliary incision that is too close to the lid margin. Finally, rounding may occur when adhesions develop between upper and lower blepharoplasty incisions that are too close.

Lower lid Hyperpigmentation and Scarring

Although discoloration can occur in both the upper and the lower eyelids, it is of greater significance in the lower eyelids because it may accentuate the "tired look" that patients complain about. Discoloration of the lower eyelid can be preexisting and related to familial traits, chronic allergies or rhinosinusitis, or shadowing related to prominent tear troughs. This should be identified preoperatively and pointed out to the patient so it is less of an issue postoperatively. Areas in which skin has been undermined are frequently evidenced by hyperpigmentation in the early recovery period secondary to bleeding beneath the skin surface with hemosiderin deposition. This process is usually self-limiting but often takes longer to resolve in darker-skinned individuals (Fitzpatrick type III and darker). It is imperative during the healing process, especially in darkly-pigmented individuals, that they avoid direct sunlight because this could lead to permanent pigment changes. Refractory cases that persist after 2 months may be considered for camouflage, periorbital peeling, or depigmentation therapy (e.g., hydroxyquinone, kojic acid). Telangectasias may develop after skin undermining, particularly in areas beneath or near the incision, and most commonly occur in patients with preexisting telangectasias or thick sebaceous skin. Options for correcting these problems may include light-based therapies, laser and chemical peeling.

Suggested Readings

1. Flowers RS. The art of eyelid and orbital esthetics: multiracial surgical considerations. Clin Plast Surg 1987;14:703–721.
2. Most SP, Mobley SR, Larrabee WF. Anatomy of the eyelids. Facial Plast Surg Clin North Am 2005;13: 487–493.
3. Doxanas MT, Anderson RL. Oriental eyelids: an anatomic study. Arch Ophthalmol 1984;102:1232.
4. Sires BS, Saari JC, Garwin GG, Hurst JS, Van Kuijk FJ. The color difference in orbital fat. Arch Ophthalmol 2001;119:868.
5. Pak J, Putterman AM. Revisional eyelid surgery: treatment of severe postblepharoplasty lower eyelid retraction. Facial Plast Surg Clin North Am 2005;13:561–569.

6. Rankin BS, Arden RL, Crumley RL. Lower eyelid blepharoplasty. In Papel ID (ed). Facial Plastic and Reconstructive Surgery, 2nd ed. New York, Thieme, 2002, pp. 196–207.
7. Quatela VC, Ries WR. Aesthetic facial surgery. In Krespi YP, Ossoff RH (eds). Complications in Head and Neck Surgery. Philadelphia, WB Saunders; 1993, pp. 385–435.
8. Baylis HI, Goldberg RA, Groth MJ. Complications of lower blepharoplasty. In Putterman AM (ed). Cosmetic Oculoplastic Surgery, 3rd ed. Philadelphia, WB Saunders, 1999, pp. 429–456.
9. Peak DA. Acute Orbital Compartment Syndrome. eMedicine online
10. Adamson PA, Constantinides MS. Complications of blepharoplasty. Facial Plast Surg Clin North Am 1995;3:211–221.
11. Rohrich RJ, Coberly DM, Fagien S, et al. Current concepts in aesthetic upper blepharoplasty. Plast Reconstr Surg 2004;113:32e–42e.
12. Lowry JC, Bartley GB. Complications of blepharoplasty. Surv Ophthalmol 1994;38:327–350.
13. Patipa M, The evaluation and management of lower eyelid retraction following cosmetic surgery. Plast Reconstr Surg 2000;106:438–453.
14. Gausas RE. Technique for combined blepharoplasty and ptosis correction. Facial Plast Surg 1999;15: 193–201.
15. Weinfeld AB, Burke R, Codner MA, The comprehensive management of chemosis following cosmetic lower blepharoplasty. Plast Reconstr Surg 2008;122:579–586.
16. Glavas IP. The diagnosis and management of blepharoplasty complications. Otolaryngol Clin North Am 2005;38:1009–1021.
17. McCollough EG, Garcia RE. Transcutaneous lower eyelid blepharoplasty with fat excision. Arch Facial Plast Surg 2006;8:374–380.
18. Perkins SW, Dyer WK Jr, Simon F. Transconjunctival approach to eyelid blepharoplasty. Arch Otolaryngol Head Neck Surg 1994;120:172–177.
19. McCord CD Jr, Shore JW. Avoidance of complications in lower lid blepharoplasty. Ophthalmology 1983; 90:1039.
20. Edgerton MT Jr. Causes and prevention of lower lid ectropion following blepharoplasty. Plast Reconstr Surg 1972;49:367.
21. McCord CD Jr. The correction of lower lid malposition following lower lid blepharoplasty. Plast Reconstr Surg 1999;103:1036.
22. Bartley GB. The differential diagnosis and classification of eyelid retraction after blepharoplasty. Ophthalmology 1996;103:168.
23. Rees TD. Prevention of ectropion by horizontal shortening of the lower lid during blepharoplasty. Ann Plast Surg 1983;11:17.
24. Kim JK, Ellis DS, Stewart WB. Correction of lower eyelid retraction by transconjunctival retractor excision and lateral eyelid suspension. Ophthalmic Plast Reconstr Surg 1999;15:341.
25. Gunter JP, Hackney FL. A simplified trans-blepharoplasty subperiosteal cheek lift. Plast Reconstr Surg 1999;103:2029.
26. De Paiva CS, Cehn Z, Koch DD, et al. The incidence of risk factors for developing dry eye after myopic LASIK. Am J Ophthalmol 2006;41:438–445.
27. Drenser SC, Saadat D. Safety of Blepharoplasty in patients with pre-operative dry eyes. Arch Facial Plast Surg 2004;6(2):101–104.
28. Michaeli A, Slomovic AR, Sakhichand K et al. Effect of Laser in situ Keratonileusis on tear secretion and corneal sensitivity. J Refract Surg 2004;20(4):379–383.
29. Carter SR, Stewart JM, Khan J, et al. Infection after blepharoplasty with and without Carbon Dioxide Laser resurfacing. Ophthalmology 2003;110:1430–1432.

10

Aesthetics of the Brow

Stephen Smith, Jr., MD, Sumit Bapna, MD, and
Edwin F. Williams, III, MD

The concepts of facial beauty have been pursued through the ages. The art and writings throughout the history of civilization confirm this. As every era, culture, and ethnicity might define beauty differently, the facial plastic surgeon may be challenged to define this elusive ideal. However, despite the varying perceptions of beauty, there are concepts that do remain steadfast, and most would agree that there is beauty in youth. An effort to restore a youthful appearance is a major goal of aesthetic surgery, and for most patients "rejuvenation" is their reason for seeking a cosmetic procedure.

Although efforts at rejuvenation have often focused on the lower face and neck, it is critical not to ignore the complex of the forehead, brow, and eyes. The upper third of the face is an area of intense focus in human interaction and should not be neglected in the pursuit of rejuvenation. To optimize our results and patient satisfaction as facial plastic surgeons, we must consider this complex and may need to educate our patients with regard to its importance.

Aging of the upper third of the face is primarily a result of gravity and a loss of elastic tissue support secondary to collagen changes in the dermis. This leads to brow ptosis, which can give a crowded or angry appearance to the eye and brow complex. Most drastically, ptotic forehead skin can present as lateral hooding over the upper eyelids. Repeated pull on the skin of the underlying facial mimetic muscles combined with the age-related laxity of the skin causes the aging brow and forehead to also display rhytides. In order for the facial plastic surgeon to address the aging forehead, the anatomy, the aesthetics of the orbital complex and brow, as well as the mechanisms of aging must thoroughly be understood (**Figure 10-1**).

Anatomy

A detailed knowledge of anatomy is required to understand the aesthetics of the brow and how it is affected with aging. The layers of the scalp are the skin, subcutaneous tissue, aponeurosis or galea, loose areolar tissue, and the periosteum. The galea is a tendinous inelastic sheet that connects the frontalis muscle to the occipitalis muscle. Laterally, the galea merges with the temporoparietal fascia. The muscles that act upon the forehead and brow include the frontalis, corrugator supercilii, procerus, and orbicularis oculi muscles. These muscles are innervated by the frontal and zygomatic branches of the facial nerve and are responsible for elevation and depression of the brow (Table 10-1). The sparse subcutaneous tissue of the forehead allows the

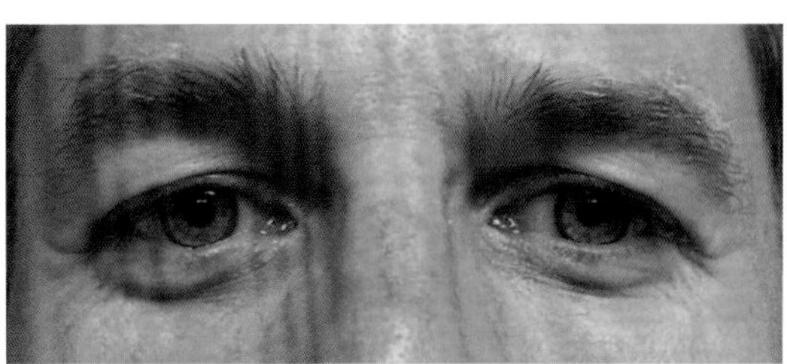

Figure 10-1. Example of brow ptosis and lateral hooding on an aged male brow.

TABLE 10.1 Classification and Function of the Muscles of the Forehead.

Muscle	*Classification*	*Function*
Frontalis	Elevator	Produces total elevation of the eyebrow
Corrugator (medial part)	Elevator	Produces partial elevation of the head of the eyebrow
Orbicularis oculi	Depressor	Orbital portion produces total depression of the eyebrow
Procerus	Depressor	Depresses the medical portion of the brow and the glabellar region
Corrugator (lateral part)	Depressor	Depresses the tail of the brow

actions of the forehead muscles to be transmitted directly to the thick overlying skin. Over time the actions of these muscles produce signs of aging such as ptosis and rhytides.

Aesthetics of the Orbital Complex

Factors including age, sex, culture, ethnicity, and current fashion trends influence the aesthetics of the eyebrow. The surrounding periorbital features are also important determinants of eyebrow appearance. There is great variety in the shape, size, and position of eyebrows; however, eyebrows that are aesthetically pleasing on one face may look abnormal on another. The concept of "an ideal eyebrow" is difficult to apply universally, but the aesthetics can be understood.

Some general contributions to the aesthetics of the brow were made by an analysis by Jack Gunter in 1997. The following is a summary of the ideal brow shape and position as well as description of the open-ended oval concept of the periorbital area according to Gunter. The medial brow should be a continuation of the aesthetic dorsal line of the nose as it curves laterally on the superciliary ridge and should begin above the medial canthus between the most prominent portion of the superciliary ridge and the supraorbital arch. The inferior margin of the brow should cross the supraorbital notch and continue upward to peak somewhere between the lateral limbus and point just beyond the lateral canthus. The vertical distance from the supraorbital arch to the peak of the brow will differ depending on the curvature of the arch in that area. However, the peak should rarely be more than 10 mm above a horizontal line off the most caudal portion of the medial brow. It should be higher in women than in men. In every case the medial brow should be lower than the lateral peak (**Figure 10-2**). The periorbital area should have its own balance as well as a balance with the rest of the face. It should resemble an oval with an open lateral end. This open-ended oval consists of the eyebrow superiorly, the nasal dorsal line medially, and the nasojugal groove inferiorly that fades as it proceeds laterally. The eye should be in the center of this oval, and size of the oval should balance with the rest of the face (**Figure 10-3**).

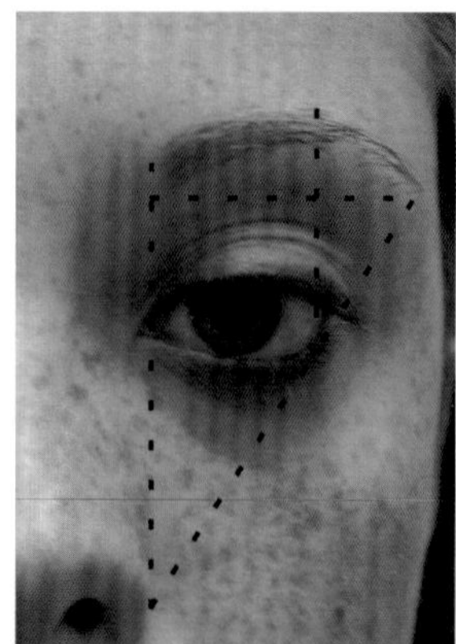

Figure 10-2. The ideal eyebrow, with the lateral peak over the area between the lateral limbus and lateral canthus.

The aesthetics of the male brow differ from that of the female brow described. The male eyebrow is positioned lower than the female brow and is typically at the level of the supraorbital rim. Additionally, the shape of the male eyebrow is less arched

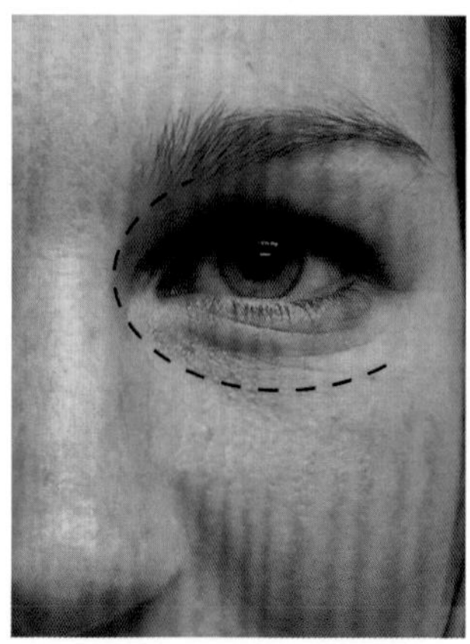

Figure 10-3. Open-ended oval concept of the periorbital area.

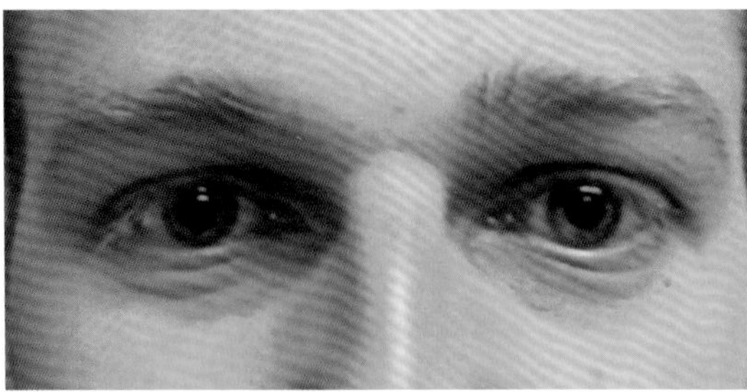

Figure 10-4. The male brow, nearly flat and overlying the supraorbital rim.

and usually flat or nearly horizontal. The lateral brow area is usually more prominent in the male, and the upper eyelid appears more masculine if fuller and slightly more redundant than in the female **(Figure 10-4)**.

The ideal shape, length, and position of the brow can also be appropriately altered to fit different shapes of faces. Most criteria of the idealized brow are based on the idealized concept of facial shape—the oval—and do not account for different facial types among individuals. There are five basic brow shapes: (1) curved, (2) sharp angled, (3) soft angled, (4) rounded, and (5) flat. Further differentiation can be made for the brow shapes in terms of the height of the arches: low, medium, and high. The oval face is intrinsically balanced and the brow plays no significant role in making the face look "more oval." Therefore, brow shape can be guided by personal taste. The round face requires lines that go up and down to make it appear more oval. A high arched brow with the peak moved out laterally accomplishes this. A round brow shape helps to add curves to soften the heart-shaped face. Flat brows will make a long face look more oval by drawing the viewer's eye from side to side instead of up and down. The square face has a strong jaw line. Strong angulated eyebrows balance this most effectively when the peak is directly over the square of the jaw. The angular diamond face shape is softened with rounded brows; also, peaked brows can help narrow the width **(Figure 10-5)**. One must look beyond generalized numbers and relationships and realize that individual characteristics of the brow and facial shape truly determine the most aesthetic brow appearance for a given person.

A more contemporary view of facial aesthetics has been described by Philip A. Young using circles of prominence. In this theory, the observer of the face fixes the most attention on the iris. All subtle shapes, sizes, and dimensions in the face are then defined by the diameter of the iris. In this model, the lateral brow should lie in the so-called first oblique

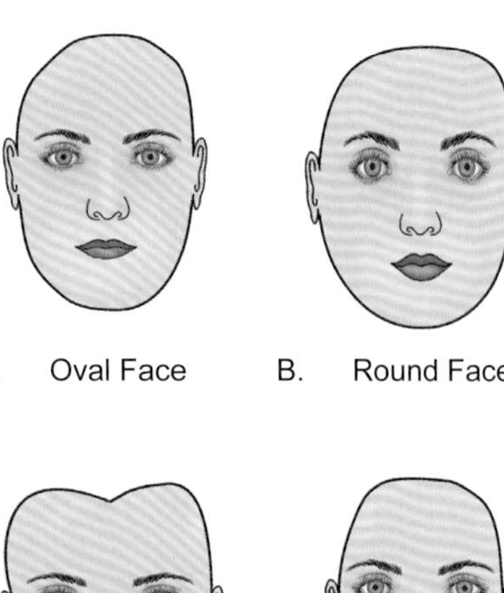

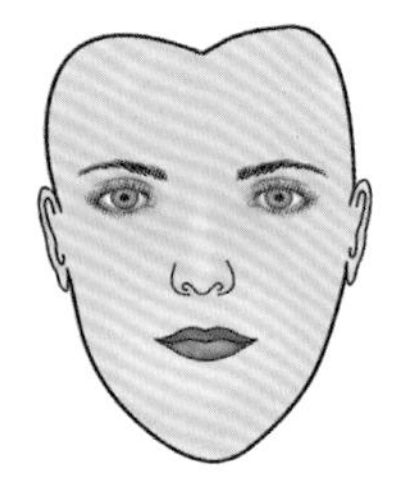

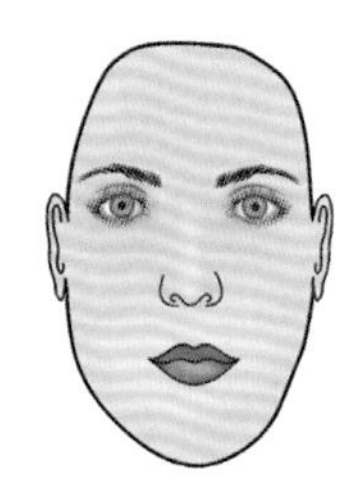

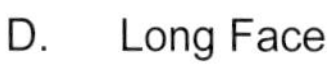

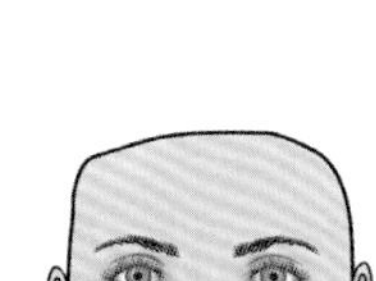

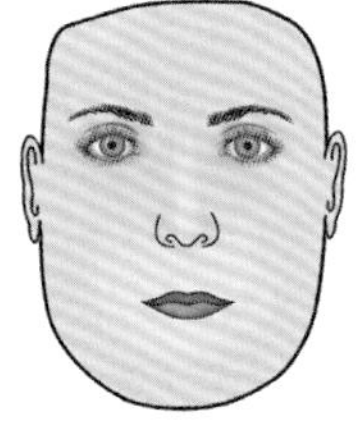

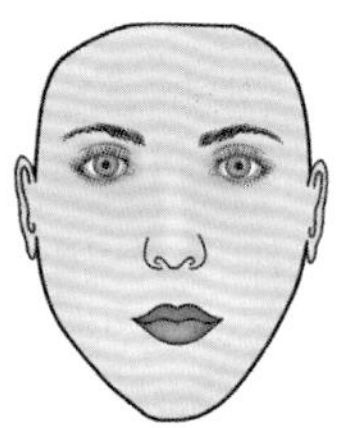

Figure 10-5. Brow shapes based on the facial shape. (a) Oval face—brow shape guided by personal taste. (b) Round face—high arched brow. (c) Heart-shaped face—round brow. (d) Long face—flat brow. (e) Square face—strong angulated brow. (e) Angular diamond face—peaked brow.

(traversing from the nasal tip through the pupil). The angle from medial to lateral brow should be 18 degrees, which is the same as the angle from the nasal tip to alae, and lower lip to commissure. The height of the eyebrow should be at most 0.5 IW (iris width) because anything greater attracts attention away from the eyes, ultimately decreasing aesthetic appeal **(Figure 10-6)**.

Mechanisms for Aging of the Brow

Three distinct deformities—brow ptosis, rhytides, and volume loss—are demonstrated in the aging forehead. All are consequences of time-related changes. Changes in the size and orientation of the elastic fibers that are responsible for maintaining

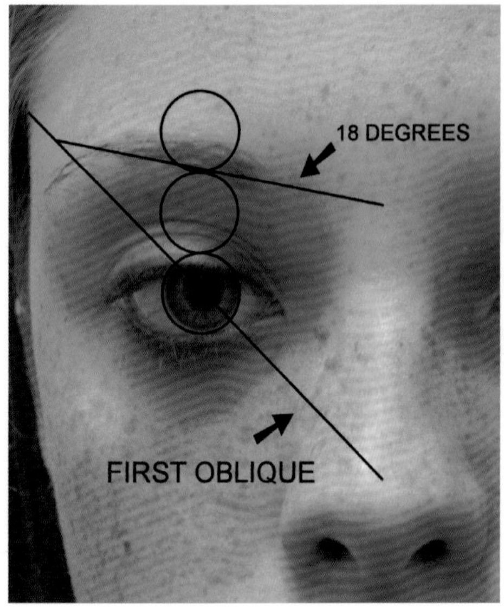

Figure 10-6. Circles of prominence theory.

skin tension, along with diminished numbers and diameter of fibers, result in a reduced dermal compliance. Brow ptosis then occurs as gravity acts on less elastic skin and decreased subcutaneous tissue. The lateral brow drops more than the medial brow.

Rhytides arise from the repeated action of facial mimetic muscles on the overlying skin. Over time the skin loses ground substance, and in combination with time-related elastolysis and collagen rearrangement, the skin becomes more prone to wrinkling. Horizontal forehead creases are caused by the action of the frontalis muscle. The vertical glabellar furrows are caused by the action of the corrugator supercilii muscle and the procerus muscle causes the horizontal glabellar furrows.

Patient Evaluation

The surrounding features of the face need to be considered to adequately address the upper third of the face. This includes the location and density of the hairline, the color and thickness of the forehead skin, and the degree of ptosis. The hairline frames the brow, and there are differences that in the male and female patient that should be recognized. The male hairline may have temporal peaks, whereas the female will usually have a rounder hairline. This shape distinction as well as the density of the hairline will influence the possible rejuvenation techniques. The degree of ptosis can be judged

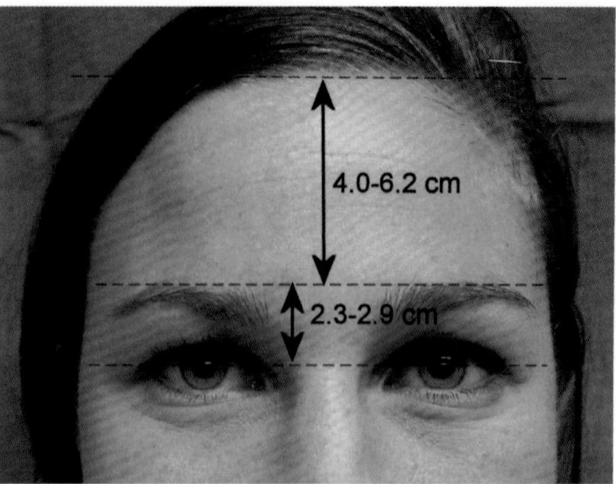

Figure 10-7. Normative values for the brow and forehead.

subjectively in an effort to create balance of the face; however, there are some quantitative measures that can be applied as well. From averages determined by McKinney et al., the average distance from the top of the brow to the hairline was 4.8 cm (range of 4.0–6.2 cm) and the distance from the top of the brow to the midpupil was 2.5 cm (range of 2.3–2.9 cm). As mentioned previously these "normative" values (**Figure 10-7**) should be used a simple guideline with the primary goal of balance and harmony. Other important preoperative details of brow rejuvenation include photographic documentation and recognizing eyelid problems, such as blepharoptosis, blepharochalasis, lid ptosis, and lagophthalmos.

Conclusion

The brow is an important component of the beautiful face. To address the aging forehead and brow completely, the aesthetic analysis and anatomy of the region must be studied carefully. The facial plastic surgeon has many tools to address this area, from minimally invasive modalities, such as botulinum toxins and fillers, to longer lasting procedures, such as the brow lift. With aging many changes occur, disturbing the natural balance of the orbital complex and surrounding structures including the midface. Focus should be turned to this area as well because correction of the aging midface specifically allows for improvement of the lateral brow, a common complaint of the aging face patient. In summary, rejuvenation techniques for the brow should rarely occur in isolation; the midface and periorbital structures are intimately linked and should be dealt in concert with the brow.

Suggested Readings

1. Koch JR, Troell RJ, Goode RL. Contemporary management of the aging brow and forehead. *Laryngoscope* 1997;107(6):710–715.
2. Gunter JP, Antrobus SD. Aesthetic analysis of the eyebrows. *Plast Reconstr Surg* 1997;99(7):1808–1816.
3. Alex JC. Aesthetic considerations in the elevation of the eyebrow. *Facial Plast Surg* 2004;20(3):193–198.
4. Young PA, Sinha U, Rice DH, Stucker F. Circles of prominence: A new theory on facial aesthetics. *Arch Facial Plast Surg* 2006;8:263–267.
5. Presti P, Yalamanchili H, Honrado CP. Rejuvenation of the aging upper third of the face. *Facial Plastic Surgery*. 2006;22(2):91–96.
6. Conner MS, Karlis V, Ghali GE. Management of the aging forehead. *Oral Surg Oral Med Oral Pathol* 2003;95(6):642–648.
7. Knize DM. An anatomically based study of the mechanism of eyebrow ptosis. *Plast Reconstr Surg* 1996;97(7):1321–1333.
8. McKinney P, Mossie RD, Zukowski ML. Criteria for the forehead lift. *Aesthet Plast Surg* 1991;15(2):141–147.
9. Byrd HS, Burt JD. Achieving aesthetic balance in the brow, eyelids, and midface. *Plast Reconstr Surg* 2002;110(3):926–933.

Index

Note: Page references with *f* indicate figures; page references with *t* indicate tables.

52检